More
Than a
Place

More Than a
Than a
Place

The Origins of a
Children's Hospital at Vanderbilt

Lisa A. DuBois

Providence House Publishers
WWW.PROVIDENCEHOUSE.COM
FRANKLIN, TENNESSEE

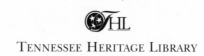

TENNESSEE HERITAGE LIBRARY

Printed in the United States of America

11   10   09   08   07   1   2   3   4   5

Library of Congress Control Number: 2007928104

ISBN: 978-1-57736-387-3

Vanderbilt University Medical Center gratefully acknowledges the Junior League of Nashville and Friends of Vanderbilt Children's Hospital for their generous support of this project. We are also most grateful to Allaire Karzon for her energy and commitment to having this story told.

Net profits and author's proceeds from the sale of *More Than a Place* benefit the Monroe Carell Jr. Children's Hospital at Vanderbilt.

Cover and page design by Joey McNair
Cover art by Diana Duren
Cover photo by Dana Johnson

A Hillsboro Press Book

Providence House Publishers
238 Seaboard Lane • Franklin, Tennessee 37067
www.providencehouse.com
800-321-5692

To Dr. David Karzon,
who figured out how to realize the dream

Contents

Illustration Credits

The author is grateful to the many individuals and organizations who graciously provided images and granted permission to include them in this book.

Photographs on pages 7–8, 36, 38, 41–42, 55, 57–58, 64, 67–68, 70–71, 74, 123, 125, 127, 136, 157, 175, 184, 186, 193, 195, 198, 200, 202, 213, 231, 240 are courtesy of Vanderbilt Historical Collection, Eskind Biomedical Library.

Photograph on page 11 is courtesy of the family of Cornelia Keeble Ewing.

Photographs on pages 15, 17, 25, 27, 29–30, 34, 90–91, 99–100, 116, 133–134, 162, 169, 186 are courtesy of the Junior League of Nashville archives.

Photographs on pages 76, 80, 82, 84, 87 are courtesy of the Archives of the Jewish Federation of Nashville and Middle Tennessee.

Photograph on page 97 is courtesy of the family of Mary Lee Manier.

Photographs on page 104, 151, 215–216, 233, 235, 246, 248 are courtesy of Vanderbilt University Medical Center Office of News and Public Affairs.

Photograph on page 149 is courtesy of the family of Dr. David and Allaire Karzon.

Photograph on page 183 is courtesy of the Jewish Federation of Nashville and Middle Tennessee.

Photograph on page 190 is courtesy of the family of William Ross.

Photograph on page 194 is courtesy of Vanderbilt Neonatal Intensive Care Department.

Photograph on page 196 is courtesy of the family of William Cook.

Photographs on page 209 are courtesy of the families of Wilson "Woody" Sims, Mary Stumb, and Fran Hardcastle.

Photographs on page 250 and 253 are courtesy of Earl Swensson Associates, copyright Hedrich Blessing.

We also acknowledge and thank the *Tennessean* for permission to reprint material and images which were originally published by that newspaper, and to which the *Tennessean* retains the copyright.

Foreword

In February 2004, with precision and coordination reminiscent of a military operation, 103 children moved from the fifth and sixth floors of the Vanderbilt Hospital to the nation's newest and best free-standing children's hospital in the world . . . the Monroe Carell Jr. Children's Hospital at Vanderbilt. It was one of the proudest days of my life and it marked the end of a chapter for Vanderbilt, for our hospital, for the patients and families we serve, and for our community.

The chapter in history that concluded on that day was written by some amazing people. It is their legacy that lives on today in the spirit that fills our new hospital. We are the embodiment of their values. They believed in offering care for every child regardless of ability to pay. They demonstrated a spirit of philanthropy. They were focused and tenacious. They firmly believed in the prospect of a better tomorrow. We are the very proud inheritors of their work and their work ethic, and for that we are deeply grateful.

This book is produced as part history and part tribute to the fascinating and devoted people who have entrusted the future of Children's Hospital to us. This is a story about a cause. It is the story of people and the things they did, great and small. It is a story about Nashville, as it struggled with some of the most tumultuous times in its two-hundred-year history. And, finally, this is a story about the pain and healing and triumph that is often brought about by change.

Dr. Harry Jacobson
Vice Chancellor for Medical Affairs
Vanderbilt University Medical Center

Preface

This book shares an episode in history that took place over the span of nearly forty years—from the time in which the citizens of Nashville began crusading for a children's hospital until Vanderbilt Children's Hospital finally emerged as a deliberate entity, a carefully planned hospital-within-a-hospital.

More Than a Place is not intended to be an historical account of Vanderbilt Medical Center, the Vanderbilt Pediatrics Department, or the Junior League of Nashville. Instead, its purpose is to provide a bird's-eye view of the confluence of forces that made the hospital happen, despite the many odds working against it. As a result, quite a few seminal events in both Nashville's and Vanderbilt's histories during the time frame under discussion may not be included here. Also, many people who may have been instrumental in the creation of the hospital may have been omitted from the text—either because of difficulty reaching them, because they didn't leave an obvious paper trail of their involvement, or because they were never mentioned by those being interviewed, who were asked to recall events that took place decades earlier. My apologies to those who may have been left out of the text, because I'm sure they would have provided additional insight and perspective to the tale.

Finally, the events presented here are rendered as accurately as possible, given the constraints of time, resources, and memory. In some cases, various people recalled the exact same events quite differently. Past occurrences and relationships are seen through the haze of distance and removal from them. Therefore, I have tried to distill the truth as best as possible from interviews, minutes of meetings, memos, historical records, and newspaper clippings. If I didn't hit the mark, please accept my apologies. It wasn't for lack of trying.

Ultimately, I hope the reader views this book as an account of a larger group of citizens from both inside and outside of Vanderbilt, who strove to do the best thing for the children of their region, even when they disagreed on what that might be. They number in the hundreds. They are all worthy of admiration for remaining dedicated to such a noble endeavor—and whether or not they made it onto the pages of this book, they deserve to be applauded for their courage and their generosity.

Acknowledgments

This book would never have been started, much less completed, were it not for a long line of people determined to see it come to fruition. First among these are Dr. David and Allaire Karzon. In the summer of 2004, they decided that I should be the writer to undertake this task, and they refused to give up until I agreed to do it. The Karzons were most generous in every respect. They opened up all their files and personal records about Vanderbilt Children's Hospital and then cut me loose to explore them as I saw fit. They are the force behind *More Than a Place*.

I was granted an author's ultimate luxury. After I was commissioned to write the book by Joel Lee, associate vice chancellor for communications at Vanderbilt University Medical Center, he let me tell the tale that I saw unfolding. He never asked that I smooth over disputes, promote the university, or make events appear less rocky or contentious than they actually had been. The same is true of the Junior League of Nashville, the Friends of Vanderbilt Children's Hospital, the Jewish Federation of Nashville, and other groups with an interest in the story. They all entrusted me with their histories, and for that I am truly appreciative.

I must also acknowledge the help given by Dr. Robert and Elizabeth Collins. Initially, I had planned to place the beginnings of the book in the late 1960s. Elizabeth Collins suggested that I would probably want to look into events that happened a good bit earlier. When I resisted, she gave me the names of former Junior League presidents Mary Louise Tidwell, Joanne Bailey, and Mary Lee Manier, and gently informed me that they would be expecting my calls. Those phone calls, which I dutifully made, opened up a whole new direction for the book. It was no longer simply about Vanderbilt or a hospital, but about an entire community of people and a decades-long debate about how to best serve the needs of area children in a changing society.

In particular, I must thank Mary Teloh, archivist for the Vanderbilt Historical Collection at the Eskind Biomedical Library. I'm also indebted to Beth Odle and the other archivists at the Nashville Room of the Nashville Public Library; Annette Ratkin, archivist at the Jewish Federation of Nashville and Middle Tennessee; John Howser and Bill Snyder, of the Vanderbilt University Medical Center Office of

News and Public Affairs; Carole Bartoo, of the Children's Hospital Office of News and Public Affairs; and Mary Lee Bartlett and Susan Moll, of the Junior League of Nashville. I also appreciate the generous assistance given by Terri Seale, Suzy Wilkinson, Ted Gilbert, Missy Scoville, and Providence House Publishers, in particular, Andrew Miller and Nancy Wise.

I couldn't be more grateful to the following people, who agreed to be interviewed, and in some cases, shared their photos, scrapbooks, and memorabilia with me: Mary Louise Tidwell, Mary Lee Bartlett, Suzy Woolrine, Dr. Stuart Finder, Mary Lee Manier, Joanne Bailey, Liza Lentz, Nelson Andrews, Ridley Wills, Irene Wills, Dr. Ian Burr, Dr. Thomas Graham, Frances Jackson, Mary Stumb, Betty Nelson, Dr. Bill DeLoache, Nickie Lancaster, Justine Milam, John Seigenthaler, Fran Hardcastle, Woody Sims, Dr. George Holcomb, Dr. Jim O'Neill, Joanne Nairon, Dr. Sarah Sell, Libby Werthan, William Ross, Dr. Bob Merrill, Linda Christie Moynihan, Ed Nelson, Carole Nelson, Bennie Batson, Dr. Pete Riley, Alice Hooker, Dr. Eric Chazen, Louise Katzman, Dr. Bill Altemeier, Dr. Jennifer Najjar, Dr. Bob Cotton, Kent Ballow, Suzanne Windorfer, Bill Bell, Dr. William Wadlington, Elizabeth Jacobs, Dr. John Lukens, Frances Preston, Joan Bahner, Pat Wilson, Bill Cook, Jean Cook, Dr. David Thombs, and Lewis Lavine.

Jane Tugurian's editorial skills and historical insight were invaluable, as were Ditty Abrams's line editing assistance and emotional encouragement. I must also thank Marie Griffin, Lydia Howarth, Beth Stein, and Missy Beattie for shoring me up as I went through this process.

Finally, I want to extend my deepest love and gratitude to Ethan and Shelley, and especially to Ray, who never wavered in their support for this project even when I was working some rather insane hours. I couldn't have done it without them.

Lisa A. DuBois
November 2006

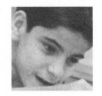

Prologue

"The edge of darkness has been pushed back . . ."

—Ed Huddleston
Nashville Banner, April 12, 1955

On April 12, 1955, *Nashville Banner* reporter Ed Huddleston arrived, notepad in hand, on the ward of Vanderbilt University Hospital often referred to as "Tank Town" or, more officially, the Regional Poliomyelitis Respiratory Center. There he quizzed victims of poliomyelitis—polio patients confined to noisy, mechanical iron lungs, crippled or paralyzed patients struggling to regain function in their arms and legs, patients for whom the news would, unfortunately, change nothing. Jonas Salk had discovered a polio vaccine that was 90 percent effective.

"What do you think of the news?" the beat writer asked ten-year-old Gayle Hines, her arms and neck wrapped in slings and pulleys attached to a special wheelchair.

"I think it's nice!" replied the little girl.

"Nobody said, 'Too late . . .' " Huddleston wrote later that day. *"Everybody said, 'Thank God! . . . the edge of darkness has been pushed back. . . .' "*

At the same moment that Huddleston was interviewing polio patients, Dr. Amos Christie, chairman of the Vanderbilt pediatrics department, was behind the wheel of his car, speeding downtown, with faculty members Dr. Randy Batson and Dr. Harris "Pete" Riley holding on for dear life. They arrived at the Noel Hotel in time to hear revered virologist Dr. Thomas Francis Jr. announce at a national press conference, "The vaccine works. It is safe, effective, and potent."

All across America people celebrated. On that day, it looked like scientists had finally broken the back of one of the most terrifying diseases known in the twentieth century. On that day, there was hope.

What individuals didn't understand and couldn't foresee was that the demise of polio would have ramifications that would spread far beyond the ward called Tank Town. The people of Nashville couldn't know that just south of downtown on White Avenue, this day would mark the beginning of profound change in which the well-heeled ladies of local society would begin a process that would ultimately force them to reexamine the definition of the "crippled child." That definition, they would conclude, must be expanded to embrace children with physical, medical, and emotional disabilities—and it must also include children of all races.

Nor could they predict that eliminating the threat of polio would sow the seeds for a confrontation that would pit the citizens of Nashville against the administration and faculty of Vanderbilt University Medical Center, one side insistent upon, and the other side resistant to, building a children's hospital in the community.

And finally, they could not predict that in upstate New York, a young scientist at the University of Buffalo Children's Hospital was celebrating this day as well. He had worked on the Salk vaccine and would continue to work on its successor, the Sabin vaccine. Years later, he would carry a vision to Nashville, and he would hold fast to that vision despite upheavals from the aftermath of the civil rights movement and the Vietnam War, through accusations from an angry faculty, as well as roadblocks thrown up by an intractable Board of Trust, who were acutely aware of the dire condition of the university's finances. He wouldn't give up until his vision—the creation of a pediatric hospital at Vanderbilt that could serve all of the children of Middle Tennessee—became a reality. Yet even he could not envision what a unifying force this hospital would become.

Meanwhile, as doctors across the country awaited the manufacture and delivery of the polio vaccine to their hospitals and clinics, American children were suddenly flush with the possibility of going to sleepover camps, swimming holes, city parks, and county fairs without fear of contracting disease. For the first time in decades, they would look forward to summer with excitement and relief, rather than dread.

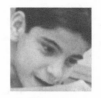

Genesis | 1

*"The intern carries a stethoscope to avoid
being mistaken for an orderly."*

**—Dr. Owen H. Wilson, MD (1870–1960),
first chairman of pediatrics at Vanderbilt School of Medicine**

On February 8, 2004, Vanderbilt University Medical Center opened up the freestanding Monroe Carell Jr. Children's Hospital at Vanderbilt to much fanfare. Community volunteers clad in yellow T-shirts lined the halls, speaking into walkie-talkies, and leading visitors on group tours. Inpatient children were transported to their new rooms on gurneys decorated with balloons and ribbons. Music played. Camera bulbs flashed. Mascots danced in the hallways. This was a momentous day for the citizens of Nashville and the surrounding counties of Middle Tennessee—the inauguration of a gleaming, 600,000-square-foot pink granite and blue glass hospital designed specifically for the needs of area children. Many people had planned, worked, and waited for nearly ten years for this dream structure, this paragon of high technology, to come to fruition.

And there were others who had waited for half a century.

This is the story of the people and events that shaped the dream begun in the 1950s, and of battles waged for twenty-five years, ending with a universal truce when the new Vanderbilt University Hospital building opened in 1980.

The founding of Vanderbilt Children's Hospital was, on the surface, unremarkable. Many cities had designated children's hospitals, some of them since the late nineteenth century. Like many other

3

children's hospitals in America, Vanderbilt's was sparked by a concerned group of local women demanding better medical care for indigent children.

What makes the genesis of Vanderbilt Children's Hospital unique is its time—the first few decades after World War II, a boom phase for research and discovery; the place—Nashville, Tennessee, a city reluctantly transforming from the Old South to the New South; and the people—a cadre of citizens driven by an unusually strong sense of civic commitment and an even stronger sense of humor.

By virtue of its physical location in the heart of the southern central United States, Nashville has always exuded a quality of self-determination. Situated by the Cumberland River in a natural basin smack dab in the center of the state, it is surrounded to the north, south, and east by the Highland Rim, and the Smoky, Blue Ridge, and Appalachian Mountains; and to the west by the Mississippi Delta. Before the start of the Civil War, Middle Tennesseans were decidedly ambivalent, siding with neither their anti-secessionist statesmen in East Tennessee, nor with their Confederate-leaning brethren in Memphis. Only after the firing on Ft. Sumter in South Carolina and President Lincoln's subsequent call to arms to stop secession did Tennesseans rally behind their pro-Unionist governor, Isham Harris. Tennessee was the last state to join the Union cause, and great numbers of young men from Tennessee enlisted on both sides of the conflict.[1]

With its rich farmlands, manufacturing centers, and sturdy rivers, Nashville had long been a thoroughfare for commerce, and naturally, a prime target for both armies. Left undefended, on February 24, 1862, the city fell to Federal soldiers and remained in Union hands for the duration of the Civil War, serving as a major supply center for the western Union command. While the city was spared the destruction wrought upon other areas of resistance, hungry armies from the Union and the Confederacy devastated its rich outlying farmlands, leaving much of post-war Middle Tennessee in a state of poverty and destitution from which it would never fully recover.[2]

Vanderbilt University was a by-product of the War between the States, founded in 1873 during Reconstruction in a tactic many consider a sleight of hand. Methodist minister Holland N. McTyeire convinced New York shipping and railroad magnate "Commodore" Cornelius Vanderbilt, a roguish tycoon who played both sides during the war, to donate half a million dollars (later ratcheting that total up to one million dollars) towards a major university in the South for training young minds and men of the cloth. The Commodore envisioned the university bearing his name as an institute for repairing the rifts left by the Civil War. McTyeire viewed it more as a vehicle for training generations of Methodist ministers.

By the turn of the century, the Vanderbilt academic administration had grown increasingly uncomfortable with the denominational restrictions demanded by its overseers. If Vanderbilt were to become a great institution, they believed, it must encourage, rather than limit, the faculty's and students' free expression and exploration into the arts and sciences. In an acrimonious 1914 divorce, the university severed its ties with the Methodist church and became a sectarian academy.[3]

The medical school at Vanderbilt University came into being before the university even had a campus. During Reconstruction, so-called medical colleges sprang up all over the country, churning out young men with medical degrees, who may or may not have sat in on the four months' worth of required coursework. One physician wrote of the low caliber of medical school enrollees as being " . . . too stupid for the bar, too immoral for the pulpit."[4]

On April 21, 1874, the medical faculty at the University of Nashville joined into an agreement with the fledgling Vanderbilt University, granting medical diplomas to students from either institution. Soon an intense rivalry brewed between the two schools as they fought over qualified students and professors. Within ten years, Vanderbilt had usurped its partner and was attracting the better faculty, staff, and students. The two medical schools parted ways in 1895.[5, 6]

That same year, Dr. Owen H. Wilson, a part-time clinical lecturer, was elected professor of anatomy at the Vanderbilt School of Medicine, and in 1905, was named the first chairman of the pediatric department.[7] Pediatrics, in that era, was not particularly different from adult medicine in terms of medical interventions. Doctors relied on comforting the child, searching for visual cues that might indicate disease, and honing their senses of touch and smell for diagnosis. In other words, pediatrics was largely nontechnological, and to some practitioners, the purest of the medical specialties.

The American system for teaching medicine, however, had become haphazard in the best cases and flat-out dangerous in others. That began to change in 1910, influenced by the release of the Flexner Report,[8] a study underwritten by the Carnegie Foundation. A secondary teacher by training, Abraham Flexner had studied the curricula and requirements of medical colleges from coast to coast and concluded that far too many of them were substandard. A great number, in fact, were beyond salvation.

According to Flexner, American medical schools needed to adhere to the tenets established by Dr. William Osler during his tenure at the Johns Hopkins School of Medicine in Baltimore. Osler insisted that all medical students must attend lectures in the classroom but also participate in practical education. He wrote:

> The art of the practice of medicine is to be learned only by experience; 'tis not an inheritance; it cannot be revealed. Learn to see, learn to hear, learn to feel, learn to smell and know by that practice alone can you become expert.[9]

Under the Oslerian model, medical students would be trained at the bedside under the mentorship of practicing physicians, gain laboratory experience by working in bacteriology labs, and, first and foremost, would treat their patients with kindness and empathy.

"The motto of each of you as you undertake the examination and treatment of a case should be 'put yourself in his place,'" Osler told a group of protégés. "Realize, so far as you can, the mental state of the patient, enter into his feelings . . . Scan gently his faults. The kindly word, the cheerful greeting, the sympathetic look."[10]

After Flexner compared the four medical colleges in Nashville, he determined that none of them met the benchmarks set by Osler, but that Vanderbilt's, at least, came the closest. As James Summerville writes, despite Vanderbilt Medical School's "lax admissions, high rate of dropouts, and foul dissecting rooms," Flexner still deemed it the best one operating in the South.[11] He named Vanderbilt, "the institution to which responsibility for medical education in Tennessee should now be left."[12]

As a result, the University of Nashville closed down its medical education department and the University of Tennessee's medical branch bounced from Nashville to Knoxville to Memphis. That left only two medical schools in Nashville—Vanderbilt and Meharry

Medical College, which the Flexner Report considered to be one of only two programs in the nation capable of training black physicians.[13]

Winding up on the plus side of the Flexner Report led to a tremendous windfall for the Vanderbilt School of Medicine. The Carnegie Foundation and other philanthropic organizations pumped cash into university coffers to ramp up its teaching and research activities. With those funds, Chancellor James Kirkland reorganized the medical school, moving it from the old downtown South Campus to a plot of land adjacent to the main campus in midtown Nashville. Finally in 1925, Vanderbilt's medical school came to rest within the bounds of the university, creating a natural environment for communication and intellectual exchange.

Beginning in the 1920s, another phenomenon swept the practice of medicine—technology. Doctors leaned more heavily on devices to help them evaluate a patient's condition. They examined X-rays for signs of tumors and malformations, and listened to patients' chests with modern stethoscopes that could distinguish between various intensities of heart and lung sounds. In time, the profession became more stringent, objective, and scientific. While new technologies led to burgeoning knowledge of the human condition in its injured and diseased states,

In the 1920s, Chancellor James Kirkland and Dean of the Medical School Canby Robinson relocated Vanderbilt University Medical School and Hospital to land adjacent to the main campus in midtown Nashville.

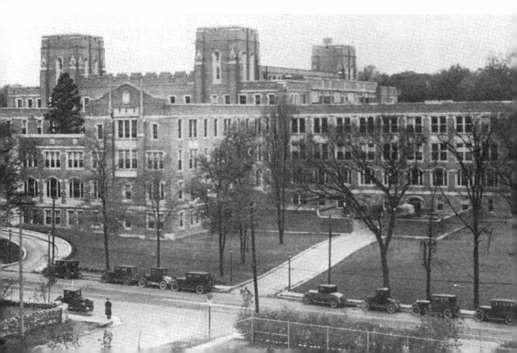

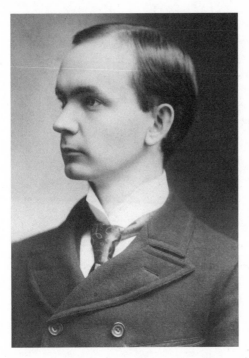

Dr. Owen Wilson was named Vanderbilt's first chairman of the Department of Pediatrics.

and subsequently, to better treatments, the practice of medicine also lapsed into something much more impersonal. Hospital walls were painted green. Doctors and nurses wore white from head to toe. The beds were hard and uncomfortable. Family members had to obey strict visiting hours and were asked to stay away from inpatients. Clinics were frighteningly sterile. Medicine became a career that appealed to stoics. What had happened to Osler's call for humanism?

Vanderbilt's Owen Wilson lamented that medicine had transformed from a trade in the healing arts to one in mechanics. "Doctors depend slavishly upon gadgets," he groused. "The intern wears a stethoscope to avoid being mistaken for an orderly."[14]

Yet the art of healing was not entirely abandoned during this period, not in Nashville at least. In 1923, a group of women had formed an organization, a kind of service sorority, and they were determined to use their time and their husbands' money to help the poorest, most vulnerable children of the community. They wanted their charges to have not only good medical care, but to enjoy (as much as possible) all the comforts of home while they recovered—comforts like books and sing-alongs, birthday parties and Sunday school, tasty food and arts and crafts.

These women were members of the Junior League, and the children they had chosen to nurture were victims of polio.

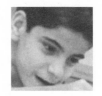

Dynamos from Dixie | 2

"People joked that if they saw my grandmother coming down the sidewalk, they'd turn and go in the other direction because they knew she'd hit them up for money. She was formidable. She was outgoing and outspoken. And she was not a beautiful woman. She looked like Eleanor Roosevelt with better orthodontia."

—Kent Ewing Ballow, granddaughter of Junior League of Nashville founder, Cornelia Keeble Ewing

In 1901, alarmed by the issues facing the swarm of immigrants streaming into Manhattan's Lower East Side neighborhoods, nineteen-year-old New York debutante Mary Harriman founded the national Junior League association. She believed that young ladies of means could join together as a group to assist the indigent with settlement problems, literacy, and nutrition.

Harriman enlisted eighty of her peers into what was specifically termed a "league" (not to be confused with a club, which might connote an exclusive girls' social gaggle). These women agreed to access the resources available to them, to get their hands dirty, and to work—for free. Among the friends she induced into activism was Eleanor Roosevelt, who as a member of the Junior League of New York taught calisthenics and dancing to young girls at the College Settlement House.[1]

Over the next twenty years, women in cities across the country began establishing local Junior League chapters. During World War I, members sold bonds and worked in military hospitals. Leagues began focusing on disparities in education. In Brooklyn, they pressured the Board of Education to provide free lunches to needy children, and the St. Louis Leaguers campaigned for voting rights for women. By the early 1920s, so many cities had established charters that a group of thirty Junior Leagues created an umbrella association (the Association of Junior Leagues of America or AJLA) to support local chapters and to ensure that the integrity of the League's mission and bylaws remained intact during an era of rapid growth.[2]

When Nashvillian Cornelia Keeble latched onto a cause, she became a warrior. In the second decade of the twentieth century, she was in her early twenties, a member of a prominent local family, and playing the characteristic role of the urbane, blue-stockinged daughter of the Deep South. She lived in an upscale home, attended the right parties, and hosted cordial luncheons. Life couldn't have been more leisurely, and Cornelia Keeble couldn't have been more restless.

In Nashville, she was surrounded by wealthy young women just like her—energetic, capable, intelligent, armed with undergraduate and graduate degrees, but with no socially acceptable outlet for their talents. Unlike many of her peers, however, Keeble had attended college in the Northeast. There she took notice as several of her friends from Philadelphia and New York discussed the selection process into the Junior Leagues of their hometowns. As members of the organization, they were required to devote substantial volunteer hours to improve the health and education of the less fortunate in their communities.

The women of Nashville, Keeble decided, could use an equivalent dose of reality. They, too, could leave their antebellum homes and wisteria-draped patios and go forth to campaign for the greater good. On April 10, 1922, with about twenty of her closest girlfriends, she formed the Nashville chapter of the Junior Leagues of America. All its members needed was a cause to ignite their passion.

World War I had ended. Men were returning from Europe maimed and broken, and the medical field faced a burgeoning demand for advances in orthopedic surgery. Even if doctors repaired shattered bones, patients and families had no idea what to do next. Few people knew which exercises were dangerous and which would aid recovery, if wounded muscles required rest or if there was a definable point when they were ready to return safely to activity.

Dr. R. Wallace Billington had opened Nashville's first orthopedic clinic at Vanderbilt in 1911, and a year later, had performed the first successful bone graft operation in the South. When war broke out, his commission sent him to the European theater where he learned the latest techniques in orthopedic surgery while simultaneously caring for injured soldiers.[3]

The city's second orthopedic surgeon, Dr. Adam Nichol, heard that the ladies of the newly formed Junior League of Nashville were considering any number of projects to undertake, and he paid them a call. What Nashville really lacked, he told them, was a place where impoverished children with polio, spinal injuries, and other orthopedic problems could convalesce. Most of these children were medically healthy, meaning they didn't have any underlying disease, but they did need a safe, hygienic, and stimulating environment in which to get well. Without long-term rehabilitation, these children had little chance of returning to a normal life. He was not interested in having the women build another cold, sterile institution, but rather something akin to a haven. If the Junior League of Nashville would underwrite such a convalescent home, Nichol proposed that he and Billington would work pro bono to deliver orthopedic care to the patients.

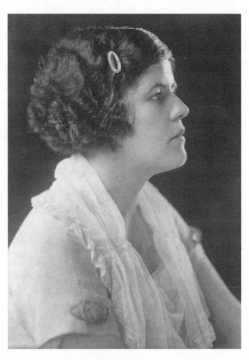

Cornelia Keeble founded the Junior League of Nashville to encourage women of privilege to volunteer to help the less fortunate in their community.

The ingredients couldn't have been more ideal— children, poverty, recovery, success. Thanks to Nichol, Cornelia Keeble and the Junior League of Nashville had found their purpose. That purpose would soon evolve into a crusade.[4]

According to its mission statement, the goal of the Junior League Home for Crippled Children was "to provide free and skilled attention to crippled children whose parents or guardians are unable to pay for such service, and whose disabilities can be sufficiently improved to enable them to be self-supporting in later life."[5]

The women faced quite a few obstacles, however. At that time, the city of Nashville had no similar type of facility. The ladies of the League would have to learn as they went along. A home for crippled children would require a building, nursing staff, special equipment, manpower, and a fairly large chunk of money to finance it. Concerned individuals warned the Junior Leaguers that they had undertaken too big a project, that as young brides and mothers they would be wiser to tackle a less daunting venture of goodwill. Polio, after all, was a contagious disease—and deadly. Untrained volunteers had no business caring for the infected offspring of strangers.[6]

Such caviling simply made the ladies all the more resolved to continue. Fortunately, Cornelia Keeble discovered a latent talent— she was, it turns out, a natural-born fund-raiser.[7]

Although she was born into and married into Southern wealth, Keeble was not the archetypal, delicate belle. Tall and big-boned, with beautiful long legs, she created a physical presence. "People joked that if they saw my grandmother coming down the sidewalk, they'd turn and go in the other direction because they knew she'd hit them up for money," said her granddaughter, Kent Ewing Ballow. "She was formidable. She was outgoing and outspoken. And she was not a beautiful woman. She looked like Eleanor Roosevelt with better orthodontia."[8]

The ladies of the Junior League began to network. They charmed their husbands and fathers into giving hefty donations. Dressed up in hats and gloves, they paid visits to local businessmen, bankers, lawyers, and merchants. They became political machines, using the clout they'd acquired as feminine legacies descended from Nashville's finest families. They even became merchants—a rummage sale added five hundred dollars to the Junior League coffers.

Nashvillians had long viewed themselves as more cultured and refined than their fellow Southerners, even dubbing their city the Athens of the South. Inspired by their success at the rummage sale, the Junior Leaguers stepped up their efforts and sponsored the renowned Viennese soprano, Maria Jeitza, to come to Nashville for a special concert. That concert netted six thousand dollars, an enormous sum in those days.

In the fall of 1923, with a little pressure and a lot of generosity, Mrs. Clyde Ezzell and the family of the late Alfred Leathers persuaded the Standard Oil Company to offer the League a building rent-free on the corner of Ninth and Monroe Street. The house could handle only nine patients at a time, but the ladies would decorate it and outfit it with all the qualities of home. Soon after, the Junior League Home for Crippled Children opened for business.[9, 10]

Since the Home employed only one staff nurse, the members assumed responsibility for the day-to-day care of the children. That meant they were in charge of such chores as helping with hygiene, changing diapers, administering physical therapy, and spoon-feeding children who were unable to feed themselves. In addition, they also kept the lawn mowed, clothes laundered, new clothes sewn, the vegetable garden tended, rooms cleaned, dishes washed, food cooked, and the boiler operational.[11, 12] Ironically, many of these women had servants to do these same chores in their own homes.

As unexpected necessities cropped up, the volunteers devoted more and more time to the Home. Said early member Mary Linda Manier Cooper, "Once, my late husband remarked that he would have to cripple our children so they could see their mother."[13]

Without knowing it, these women of the Junior League of Nashville were an integral part of a national movement towards civic responsibility. During World War I, American women had had to keep the country functional while their men were off at war. Soldiers returned home to wives and daughters who had tasted the rewards of working for higher wages in jobs typically held by men, something many found hard to give up. Even those who hadn't joined the workforce had experienced both the joys and pitfalls of sudden independence.

In Tennessee, women of social standing were particularly conflicted. Southern traditions dictated that they stay at home, raise polite children, and remain loving, attractive companions to their husbands. Yet a seminal event in 1920 had given them a new sense of empowerment. The women of Tennessee, many of them well-bred and wealthy, had engineered the final campaign that led to the passage of the Nineteenth Amendment, granting American women the right to vote.

Wisconsin and Michigan had led the charge a year earlier, and other states had fallen into place like so many dominoes. One by one male legislators had cast majority votes enabling their female citizens to vote alongside men. By August of 1920, however, the end was in sight. Both houses of the United States Congress had passed the amendment, but it needed the approval of at least thirty-six of forty-eight state legislatures to be ratified.

Because the prevailing winds indicated that the remaining states would likely block passage, suffragists (women fighting for voting rights) realized that Tennessee was their last hope, the last state with enough ambivalence in its legislature to offer the amendment a fighting chance. They persuaded Tennessee Governor A. H. Roberts to call a special session of the state General Assembly. Taken off-guard, opponents went on a slash-and-burn offensive. Historian Carole Bucy writes, "Newspaper editors portrayed 'suffs' as spinsters and 'she-males' with hen-pecked husbands."[14] In turn, the suffragists shrewdly turned a catcall about voluptuousness to their advantage. "Let us be the Perfect 36!" became their rallying cry.

Representatives from Tennessee's districts were split down the middle on the subject of ratification. The powerful liquor and rail-road lobbies were adamantly opposed to women interfering in their businesses. Factory owners in East and West Tennessee knew the suffragists would pressure them to change labor laws to benefit women and children, who were then enduring hazardous conditions working twelve-hour shifts in the textile mills. Finally, everyone knew (and some feared) that women would start raising a stink about the quality (or lack thereof) of the state's public education system.[15]

August of that year was insufferably hot and humid, fraught with muggy days and steamy nights. From states far and wide suffragists and anti-suffragists alike descended upon Nashville to wage the last great battle in the fight for voting rights. Men would cast the votes, but ultimately women would persuade them which way to turn.

Three women, Anne Dallas Dudley, Catherine Kenny, and Kate Burch Warner, led Nashville's suffragist contingent.[16] Of these, the young mother Anne Dallas Dudley—poised, beautiful, eloquent, and married to Guilford Dudley, the influential founder of the Life and Casualty Insurance Company—was chosen as the spokeswoman for the suffragists. The antis came out swinging. "Since only men can bear arms for their country, only men should vote!" they shouted.

"Yes," replied Dudley in her sweet, firm Southern drawl, "but women bear armies."[17]

By the slimmest of margins, the amendment passed. Twenty-four-year-old Harry Burns, from the tiny town of Niota in McMinn County and the youngest member of the legislature, decided at the last minute to follow his mother's advice and switched his vote in favor of ratification. Women were granted voting rights by an edge of 49 to 47.[18]

Whether they approved or disapproved of the outcome, the affluent women of Tennessee awakened to their ability to effect change, particularly when working in unity. Child labor laws passed. Education reform was brought to the table. They realized they were in a position to fight and win battles that might not alter their lives one iota—in that their children already attended the best schools, and they knew that neither they nor their friends

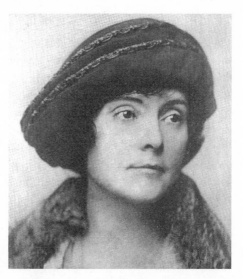

The passage of the Nineteenth Amendment in 1920 empowered local women to effect change. Suffragist Anne Dallas Dudley, here shown in the June 1926 national Junior League Bulletin, was a member of the Nashville chapter. Photo by W. S. Thuss.

would ever be forced to work in a textile mill to support their families. They could, however, profoundly benefit the underserved in their communities.

The Junior League of Nashville began to focus on the issues of the underprivileged and the less fortunate. Said Liza Beazley Lentz, "These were people who didn't have a voice. We were being their voice. That's what our Junior League does."[19]

Given the electric atmosphere of the town, the founders of the Junior League of Nashville (who were feisty even before the passage of voting rights) considered themselves unstoppable. Anne Dallas Dudley, in fact, joined the local chapter. [20] A small cadre of women, led by Cornelia Keeble and Frances Dudley Foskett Brown, traveled to Boston to attend the national conference of Junior League affiliates. While there, they asked that the next year's conference be held in Nashville. No, they were told, these conferences were always held in the Northeast. Sensing that they were being viewed as hicks from a backwater town, Brown "took the Boston Conference by storm with her 'Dynamo from Dixie' speech. . . ."[21] The executives of the national Junior Leagues were so enthralled that they selected

Nashville to host the next year's conference, the first time such a young chapter had been given such an honor.[22, 23]

While they were up north, several of the Nashville delegates went to a beauty parlor and got permanent waves put in their hair, a trendy new fashion that had not yet reached the beauticians back home.[24] The truth was, in many ways, Nashville was a backwater town.

Since the stated intention of the Junior League was an appeal to the energies and availability of youthful women, the founders understood that for the organization to have permanency, they had to establish a method for new members to come on board and for older members to age out. In keeping with that idea, Leaguers participated in tiers as either provisional, active, or sustaining members. Provisionals tended to be women in their early twenties, who were still in college or recently graduated. They were required to attend an intensive four- to six-week course for several hours three days a week. The point of provisional training was to immerse the young postulants into the tough politics and the economic disparities, as well as the social highlights, of their community. For example, a Nashville course for provisionals might include speakers ranging from judges to municipal housing authorities, from Chamber of Commerce executives to psychiatrists. They attended field trips to local theaters, hospitals, mental institutions, and charity agencies. Talks included "The Verdict Is Yours," "Industry, Planning and Government," "A City of Culture," "Our Community, Our Responsibility," and "United We Live, United We Give."[25]

After passing the provisional course, active members ranged in age from their mid-twenties until their fortieth birthday, when they became sustainers, meaning they no longer had to meet the stringent volunteer hours demanded of the younger participants. In order to keep the League at a certain size, the members held to a strict quota— they would offer invitations to only as many new members as they had active members sustaining in any one year. In other words, the process was designed to be selective and exclusive. New members had to be proposed by active members, and since their numbers were limited, each candidate was debated and voted upon by the group at large.[26]

Recalled Mary Lee Bartlett, whose mother was a Junior League member in Atlanta, "A cohort of women came to our door one afternoon. They were all decked out in their white gloves and suits and they invited my mother to become a member. And she was thrilled!"[27]

In the early days, most of the women of Nashville's League did not have jobs outside the home. The organization's heavy volunteer load prevented them from doing so, even if they'd wanted. However, Mary Louise Tidwell, daughter of newspaper owner Luke Lea, was employed as a society reporter by her father's paper, the *Nashville Tennessean*, when she was chosen to join as a provisional. Her editor gave her permission to take time off to attend the provisional course even though it cut into her work hours, on the condition that she get the inside scoop on what the well-heeled ladies in town were up to.

"You couldn't really call me a journalist, even though society reporters aspire to be Brenda Starr," Tidwell explained. "The first thing I was told was, 'All parties are lovely and all brides are beautiful. Forget the great American novel. You're writing to please!'"28

To rise as an officer in the Junior League of Nashville required dedication, a hard nose, and a thick skin. The 1929 officers are pictured below. Photo by Wiles, Nashville Tennessean, *1929.*

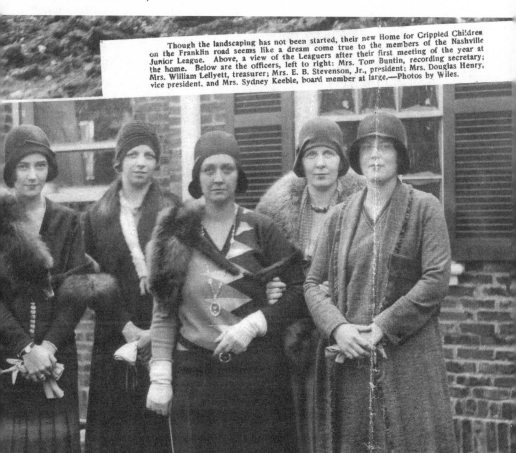

Though the landscaping has not been started, their new Home for Crippled Children on the Franklin road seems like a dream come true to the members of the Nashville Junior League. Above, a view of the Leaguers after their first meeting of the year at the home. Below are the officers, left to right: Mrs. Tom Buntin, recording secretary; Mrs. William Lellyett, treasurer; Mrs. E. B. Stevenson, Jr., president; Mrs. Douglas Henry, vice president, and Mrs. Sydney Keeble, board member at large.—Photos by Wiles.

The hallmark of the Junior League of Nashville was that its members demanded commitment. To rise in the organization and to gain influential seats on certain committees and study groups, or to be elected onto the Executive Board required dedication, a hard nose, and a thick skin. Throughout Nashville's Junior League history, nearly every president grappled with some kind of controversy, some type of trauma. As a result, while most of the city's women dreaded facing age forty, one small coterie relished the day.

As Mary Louise Tidwell prepared to assume the presidency of the local chapter in 1962, one of her predecessors, Ann McLemore Harwell, warned her how difficult her year would be. "I fell into sustaining," Harwell told her, "like a woman falls into a feather bed!"[29]

Although Junior League chapters in other cities also required members to be devoted volunteers, Nashvillians continually exceeded expectations, winning awards and setting fund-raising records. In part, this was due to the tone set early by one community power-house, Hortense Bigelow Ingram. Hortense had grown up in a wealthy family in Minnesota and in 1928, had married a Wisconsin man, Orrin Henry "Hank" Ingram, whose family had made a small fortune in the timber industry.[30] A short time later, the young married couple came to Nashville so Hank could oversee a yarn company his family had purchased shortly before the Great Depression. They liked Nashville so much that they decided to move there permanently. Hortense Ingram, however, despised the sweltering Southern summers. Therefore, every June she escaped to her family's estate in the Northeast, where she stayed until the weather back home had turned more tolerable.[31]

Within the city of Nashville lies a community known as Belle Meade. The area is noted for its stately mansions resting on impeccable yards, graced by tall magnolias, tulip poplars, silver maples, and dogwood trees. The houses face wide, manicured boulevards where cars are kept to a slow, respectable speed and people out for a stroll are required to walk in single file. To Nashvillians, Belle Meade has come to connote a social class or a specific personality, as much as a geographical location. When Hank Ingram and his bride came to Nashville, they befriended many of the people of that neighborhood and moved into the Belle Meade Apartments. Among those Hortense Ingram fell in with were ladies of the Junior League, including Cornelia Keeble, who in 1930, married prominent Nashville attorney Andrew Ewing.[32]

The Great Depression hit Tennessee hard and knocked many of the Belle Meade patriarchs, particularly those in the financial industry, for a terrible loop. Hank Ingram's business, however, weathered the Depression better than most, and he was quietly generous to his friends and colleagues in need. As a result, the Ingrams, distinctly Northerners, found themselves appreciated and accepted into the city's social circles, even though Southern lineage had always been considered a top priority.

Their daughter, Alice Ingram Hooker, said, "My parents were not brought up in the black and white [segregated] world that Nashville and the South lived with. Nor was my mother culturally or educationally in step with the attitude of the women in Nashville in the '20s and '30s, where the wife was the ornament and ran the household and enjoyed herself and was waited on like a Southern flower."[33]

Hortense Ingram was no Southern flower. Standing five-feet-two-inches tall, she was as stout as a fireplug and as direct as a lightning bolt. When it came to philanthropy, she believed that people of affluence should view it as an obligation, rather than a choice. Explained her daughter, "She thought many of her contemporaries were really oblivious to any civic responsibility. They weren't shirking something they had been told about, they had just never had that picture painted for them . . . They didn't even know they *should* be feeling that responsibility."[34]

Hortense Ingram decided she would set Nashville's upper crust straight. First, having scrutinized the landscape, she threw in her lot with the Junior League, which she deemed as having the most potential. Then she got to work by setting an example. When World War II broke out, she was one of the first women of Belle Meade to put on a uniform and work as a nurse's aide in the hospital. "She didn't just hand out coffee and doughnuts, she really went at it," her daughter said. "And she did it throughout the whole war."[35]

In addition, Hortense Ingram was as deft at mathematics and financial calculations as any man in town, garnering their sometimes grudging admiration. She was the first woman in Nashville to give one thousand dollars to the Community Chest Fund (now the United Way), setting a standard the male powerbrokers felt they, too, had to meet. Moreover, Hortense Ingram stood before the provisionals of the Junior League each year and instilled in them that hand-in-hand with their good fortunes came accountability. She expected them to invest in their local universities, hospitals, charities, and schools. They were destined to be women of action, to sit on boards, and become respected decision-makers. Rather than throwing money at local problems, they had to become involved, to devote time and effort, and to donate at levels high enough to fix those problems.[36]

Junior League member Mary Schlater Stumb had been childhood friends with the Ingram daughters. "Frankly, Mrs. Ingram scared me to death," she said. "But she taught a lot of people in Nashville how to give. She taught all of us that you need to give back to your community."[37]

Thus, the stage had already been set when the Shriners of the Al Menah Temple volunteered to help the Junior League raise the ante. In short order, the Shriners and members of the Junior League would form a bond that would last for decades; working as a team, they would begin to generate some serious capital for the Crippled Children's Home.

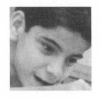

Al Menah Shriners Pitch In   3

"It was early. You would try to hit every door before people had gone to church. And you'd go door-to-door, street-by-street. Poor areas, wealthy areas, it didn't matter. No one escaped."

—Fran Hardcastle, Junior League member speaking about the Palm Sunday Paper Sale

Buoyed by their first year's success at raising money but aware that they couldn't sponsor a famous soprano every year, the women of the Junior League of Nashville began to develop novel approaches to fund-raising. What they needed was an annual event that would provide substantial, steady income on a regular basis. Intimately familiar with the mores of their city, they knew two things: newspapers were their most powerful conduits for spreading the word about the Crippled Children's Home, and Nashville's two major newspaper publishers—Major Edward Bushrod Stahlman of the *Nashville Banner* and Colonel Luke Lea of the *Nashville Tennessean*—were longtime political enemies. It might behoove them, the ladies realized, to stir up a friendly competition between the rival publications on behalf of little children suffering from polio.

In 1924, the local Junior League chapter entered into an arrangement with the *Nashville Banner*. Members went to local businesses and to friends and family in high places and sold advertisements for a special edition of the paper, receiving a percentage of the income from the ads. In addition, they collected all proceeds from the street sales of the special edition. Enthusiastic Leaguers stood on street corners, hawking their issue, blocking off Belle Meade Boulevard, and ultimately netting fifty-five hundred dollars for the Home.

For the next several years, the Junior Leaguers continued this fund-raising tactic, sometimes negotiating with the *Banner* and other years with the *Tennessean* for the privilege of subsidizing the special edition.[1, 2]

As if the stakes weren't high enough, women from both the Stahlman and Lea families participated in the Junior League. Luke Lea loaned the grateful ladies a home he owned, which they converted into the League's first clubhouse; it contained a shop, tearoom, and clubrooms.[3]

A few years afterward, Major Stahlman died and his thirty-seven-year-old grandson James G. "Jimmy" Stahlman took over as the *Banner's* president and publisher. Not insignificantly, Jimmy Stahlman had already joined the Vanderbilt University Board of Trust and would remain on the board until his death nearly fifty years later. Stahlman belonged to the Al Menah Shrine Temple, which was then an elite semi-secret society for Nashville men.[4] Luke Lea might have donated property, but Jimmy Stahlman would exercise his own clout with the blue-blooded women in town. He brought in the Al Menah Shriners to help the Junior League with their street sales of the special edition of the *Banner*.

The Shrine of North America had been founded in 1872 by thirteen men from Manhattan bent on a mission of fun and fellowship. The co-instigators of the secret order were both master showmen. Billy Florence was a handsome stage star who toured the world, playing to capacity audiences. Dr. Walter Fleming, a practicing New York physician and surgeon, "could have earned a good living as a juggler and magician."[5] While the two were becoming fast friends and discussing how to form a new kind of social fraternity, Florence happened to attend a party in France, followed by similar parties in Cairo and Algiers, in which the guests were treated to "something in the nature of an elaborately staged musical comedy." As the performance ended, the guests became members of a secret society.[6]

Based on the notes Florence had taken about the parties, Fleming adapted a set of rituals, costumes, emblems, and symbols that would designate a new society, the Ancient Arabic Order of the Nobles of the Mystic Shrine (whose rearranged initials, not coincidentally, spell out "A MASON.")[7] While participating in private and community Shrine activities, members would don a rectangular-shaped, red-tasseled headdress, known as a fez. The fez soon became an identifier for members of the Shrine organization just as a white lab coat might be for a physician or a yellow hardhat for a construction worker.

For forty-two years, Middle Tennessee did not have its own Shrine charter, although any number of Nashville men had joined temples in Memphis, Chattanooga, and out-of-state orders. In 1912, however, a team of 32nd Degree Scottish Rite Masons and Knights Templar from Middle Tennessee organized into the Al Menah Shrine Temple (now called the Al Menah Shriners), and a year later formed the nexus of the 131st Shrine Temple in North America.[8]

In the interim between the founding of the national organization and the creation of the Middle Tennessee chapter, the Shriners of North America expanded their focus. Although members still enjoyed a healthy dose of revelry, they were also searching for an official charity to support. In 1920, the Imperial Potentate, Freeland Kendrick of the Lu Lu Temple in Philadelphia, hit upon an idea. Given the devastation caused by polio, the 364,000 members of his society could channel some of their unbridled energy toward establishing hospitals for crippled children.[9] The first Shriners Hospital opened in 1922, treating free of charge (as all the Shriners Hospitals have) crippled or burned pediatric patients up to the age of eighteen. The year before, a group of Shriners had approached Chancellor Kirkland and a group of Vanderbilt physicians about selecting a site for a one-million-dollar hospital for crippled children.[10] The Shriners never built a hospital in Tennessee; however, and the closest facility was (and is) the Shriners Hospital for Crippled Children in Lexington, Kentucky. The Lexington hospital served the areas of Kentucky, West Virginia, Ohio, Indiana, and Tennessee.[11]

Since there was no local competing facility, Nashville's Al Menah Shriners threw their support behind the Junior League's Home for Crippled Children with the blessing of the Shriner national organization—at least, initially.

The Al Menah Shriners of Tennessee brought unprecedented horsepower to the Junior League fund-raiser. There were nearly twenty-five-hundred members spread across thirty-seven counties of Middle Tennessee, with an ambassador in each county to oversee the street sales. Suddenly, the League's paper sales more than tripled to $32,024.[12, 13]

In addition to the Shriners, Stahlman shared some of his business savvy with the Junior League. He informed them that the one day that newspapers sold the most copies, and when Nashvillians were most likely to read their morning or afternoon dailies, was Palm Sunday, the Sunday before Easter. Shortly, the special edition fund-raiser became known throughout the area as the Palm Sunday Paper Sale.

By 1928, the Junior League building on Monroe Street was bursting at the seams with patients, having unfortunately outlived its usefulness. The membership set out to raise funds for a new custom-made convalescent home. They purchased five acres on White Avenue off Franklin Road and launched another fund-raising campaign, soliciting the people of Nashville for help. Within two months, they had raised fifty thousand dollars, which they pooled with a twenty-five-thousand-dollar allocation from the state of Tennessee and another twenty-five thousand dollars from their own coffers. On January 1, 1930, they enthusiastically opened a new one-hundred-thousand-dollar, state-of-the-art Junior League Home for Crippled Children with all the formality and ceremony of a good Southern christening.[14]

The Junior League of Nashville was on a roll. They had a well-financed, spanking new facility for the crippled children of the area. Thanks to the Shriners, they had a broad fund-raising network for their special edition advertisements. Plus, they had the local power-brokers tripping over themselves to gain the League's approval.

Then the Great Depression hit. Businesses cut back on advertising. In the early 1930s, newspaper publisher Luke Lea ran into financial and legal trouble after several of his business deals in North Carolina went sour. By 1933, the *Tennessean* was placed under federal receivership, and four years later, was sold at auction to Texas newsman Silliman Evans Sr., an ardent champion of Franklin D. Roosevelt and New Deal liberalism. Evans's political leanings provided a sharp contrast to Jimmy Stahlman's arch conservatism. Despite their opposing editorial stances, Evans convinced Stahlman that given the dire economy, they'd be wise to enter into a joint operating agreement to reduce costs. Both papers moved their offices to 1100 Broadway. Under the agreement, the *Tennessean* would cease publication of its evening edition and the *Banner* would stop printing its Sunday edition. From that point on, the two papers would share printing presses, circulation offices, and advertising, but would remain split by an increasingly prickly ideological divide.[15, 16, 17]

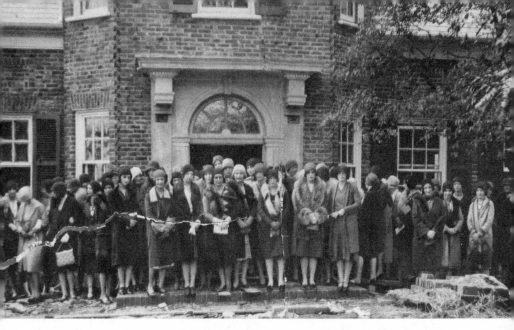

Members of the Junior League of Nashville raised enough money to build a new Home for Crippled Children on White Avenue. Photo by Wiles. Nashville Tennessean, 1929.

Hardly any debatable issue escaped argument. Wrote journalist Leon Alligood in 1998:

> If anyone suspected the vigilance of editorial protection at each newspaper, all suspicion was soon removed in what became known as the 'clock' dispute. One side of the sign outside the building identified the *Tennessean*, while the other side advertised the *Banner*. Each side had a large clock.
>
> Stahlman did not support Daylight Savings Time. Silliman Evans . . . supported it. For years Broadway drivers drove into town on Daylight Savings Time and went home on standard time.[18]

An offshoot of the joint operating agreement was that the future of the Junior League's biggest moneymaker hung in the balance. The Palm Sunday edition had become a *Banner* trademark. John Seigenthaler's uncle was the circulation director for both papers and sat in on the negotiations in which the two news mavens ironed out the finer details of their contract. According to reports, Stahlman said to Evans, "There's one thing I wish you would keep, and that's the Palm Sunday Paper Sale."

"I'm very glad to have it," Evans replied.[19]

With that exchange, the *Tennessean* inherited the Palm Sunday Paper Sale, and innocently enough, dove into an intense relationship with the Junior League that would prove to be both exhilarating and exasperating.

Although the Depression was ending, World War II soon created a paper shortage. Evans realized it was too costly for the *Tennessean* to publish an annual special issue and concluded that he would have to end the Palm Sunday tradition. Out of the despair emerged an inspiration. The Junior Leaguers negotiated with Evans to publish not a special edition, but a special tabloid, a pull-out section of the paper. This would feature heartwarming pen-and-ink illustrations of crippled children on crutches and in wheelchairs, with leg braces and neck supports, all smiling, all happy, and all in need of charitable dollars. The Junior League ladies and the Shriners would fan out across forty-one counties and walk door-to-door selling these tabloids, asking the citizens of Middle Tennessee to donate what they could afford.

Cornelia Keeble Ewing, now a senior member of the League, was certain the people of Tennessee would respond. It was an honor, she believed, to support one's community. "She had a strong sense that everybody should give back at whatever level they were capable of giving back. Not just the wealthy, but everybody," said her granddaughter Kent Ballow. "And she was just as gracious and gave just as much praise to the person struggling to make ends meet who gave two dollars or twenty dollars, as the person who made a two-thousand-dollar gift or a twenty-thousand-dollar gift. She was equally sincere in thanking them all."[20]

Cornelia Ewing's hunch was right. The Palm Sunday pull-out section became a local sensation. Shriners and Leaguers would gather at meeting places, usually participating banks, at four in the morning, collect the tabloids, and hit the streets. Some would form roadblocks on busy intersections or post themselves in the parking lots of local supermarkets and churches. Others would canvass neighborhoods on foot, ringing doorbells to awaken groggy-eyed homeowners who might be willing to dig into their pockets for a worthy cause.

League member Fran Hardcastle said:

> Girls would be assigned to Shriners. And it was early. You would try to hit every door before people had gone to church. And you'd go door-to-door, street-by-street. Poor areas, wealthy areas, it didn't matter. No one escaped. And while you would feel bad about asking some people for money, you found that people wanted to feel like

they, too, were supporting the Home. You might get a handful of change. It wasn't the money as much as them feeling like they were supporting something important to them.[21]

Middle Tennessee is notoriously hilly. Houses in many neighborhoods are spread apart on one-, two-, or five-acre lots, so going door-to-door in satellite communities like West Meade, Hillwood, Oak Hill, or Forest Hills usually meant traipsing for several miles. This was no leisurely stroll. The Junior League women enlisted their husbands, brothers, children, nieces, and nephews to join them in their Sunday morning quests. Because no neighborhood was exempt, the Palm Sunday Paper Sale also gave many young Nashvillians their first exposure to life in the poorer socioeconomic areas of the city.

The Shriners, renowned for their ability to party, made the most of these early morning crusades. Any number of them kept an emergency supply of Jack Daniel's whiskey nestled among the stacks of papers in the trunks of their cars. When they drove back to their

The Shriners of the Al Menah Temple joined with the women of the Junior League to make the Palm Sunday Paper Sale one of the biggest door-to-door fund-raisers in the country. Tennessee Governor Frank Clement and First Lady Lucille Clement (front row, fourth and fifth from right) were supporters.

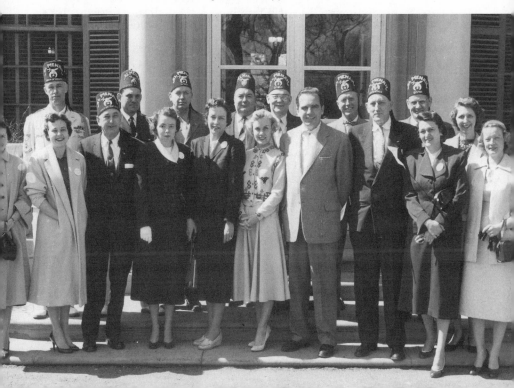

assigned headquarters several hours later, abuzz with good cheer, they carried a much lighter load.

The Palm Sunday Paper Sale became as much about publicity for the Home as it did about raising money. In fact, Junior Leaguers garnered the bulk of the donations in an Advance Paper Sale, in which they would finesse major corporate gifts from Nashville businesses. They also began a tradition of holding a Shrine Club luncheon on the Wednesday before Palm Sunday, during which they would auction off the first edition of that year's tabloid to the highest bidder. Executives soon engaged in lively philanthropic one-upmanship. The next day, the Shriners would hold a pep rally in tribute to the hundreds of people who would be out selling the next day.[22] Over time, the paper sale would generate upwards of two hundred thousand dollars a year for the Home.

The Palm Sunday Paper Sale had another purpose—it helped Shriners in outlying counties locate and identify children who might benefit from the resources available at the Home in Nashville. In many impoverished rural areas, children who had suffered and survived the crippling effects of polio, scoliosis, or juvenile arthritis spent their remaining days as invalids and/or shut-ins, with no physical or occupational therapy, schooling or job training. On their door-to-door excursions, the Shriners and Junior League ladies often made a successful pitch to the families to send these children to the Home for rehabilitation.

Said former patient Mary Ann Johns, "I was almost dead. Somehow the Junior League ladies go out into the counties and find children who are sick. Miss Eva Hagen came and found me and realized I was going to die."[23]

As a result of such rescues, the Junior League Home for Crippled Children became a landmark institution and a source of pride for citizens all across Middle Tennessee.

As the reputation of the Junior League Home for Crippled Children spread, people far and wide began including it in their wills. In order to adhere to the specific wishes of the deceased, the League needed to keep money from bequests separate from money raised at the paper sale. Members established the Endowment Trust Fund in 1940 so they could use the interest generated by bequests for the purposes stated by the donors. They also formed a Home Administration Board, apart from the Executive Board, to oversee all the operations of the Home.[24]

In most cases, the money from the Trust was deposited and allocated smoothly, because the Home Board committee worked meticulously to stay on the straight and narrow. However, the Trust did hit several snags. Sometimes interest from the Trust grew so rapidly and created such a big surplus that League members had difficulty meeting the demands set by the will. For example, one donor established a fund specifically to "gladden the hearts of children at Christmas."

"You finally ran out of things you could do with a certain amount of money!" explained former Home Board Chair Frances Jackson. "I think at one point we tried to enlarge 'Christmas' to encompass New Year, Easter, birthdays. . . ."[25]

At other times, the League received bequests from rural, semi-illiterate people. On a piece of plain white paper, in scratchy handwriting, they might have stated that they wanted some portion of their estates to go to "crippled children." On several occasions, relatives who'd been left out of the wills contested them, arguing, for example, that the term "crippled children" was not an automatic reference to the patients at the Junior League Home in Nashville. Given the lack of young invalids in the immediate vicinity, these relatives felt that they were entitled to the inheritance.

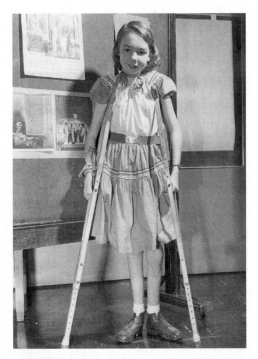

The Palm Sunday Paper Sale also served as an outreach to children from outlying counties who needed treatment and were brought in to the Junior League Home for convalescence.

Why would relatives of cash-poor farmers file lawsuits against a reputable charitable group like the Junior League of Nashville? The answer is that Tennessee was growing, and undeveloped property was extremely valuable. In some cases, rural estates amounted to several hundred acres of prime farmland or coveted suburban plots. Farming tools left to the Home could be worth thousands of dollars.[26] The Junior League won these lawsuits and the Trust blossomed into a substantial endowment.

In its new quarters, the Junior League Home for Crippled Children was able to expand its staff, employing a superintendent, a full-time physiotherapist, and a licensed teacher furnished by the county Board of Education. Thirteen local physicians, primarily orthopedists and pediatricians, rotated through the facility on a pro bono basis, with the assistance of two nurses and three nurses aides. Later, recreation and occupational therapists would join the staff. In 1938, the Home opened an outpatient clinic for children who did not require residential care.[27, 28]

The Home had a bed capacity of forty children, ranging in age from birth to fourteen years old (later increased to fifty beds and including children up to sixteen years old). They rose at 7:00 a.m.,

No matter the disability, all children at the Home were required to continue their schoolwork. Photo by Howard Cooper.

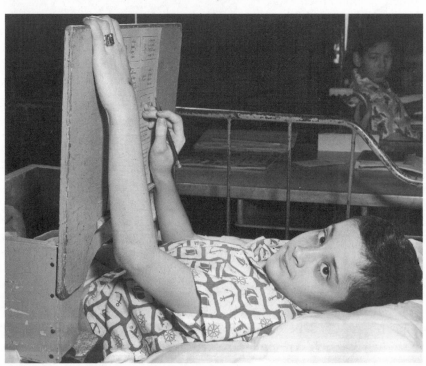

began school at 8:30 a.m., then went to physical therapy sessions, which were followed by lunch, an afternoon snack of milk, a recreation hour, dinner, and a bath. Bedtime was 7:00 p.m. sharp.[29] At least, no one at the Junior League Home suffered from a lack of routine.

Nickie Lancaster was paralyzed by polio at age eight, and after a bone graft and spinal fusion operation several years later, was fitted with a total body cast that kept her left arm out and extended. "At the Junior League Home, they rolled you into the classroom, bed and all. I was out of school for three years, but I didn't miss a single year of school[ing] here," she said. "The state of Tennessee made a valiant effort to ensure that handicapped children were educated. That's why so many polio patients had a post-high school education."[30]

For many patients, the Home provided a wonderful environment and a safe place to recover from a devastating illness. In keeping with the feeling at the time that outside influences upset the children, parents were allowed to visit only on weekends. Because many families didn't own cars, some had to travel long distances by bus to get there. Others were completely overwhelmed by the problems of transportation and home obligations, so they didn't see their children for months on end. To enliven the atmosphere at the Home, League members threw birthday and holiday parties for the children. They drove them by station wagon to local clinics when medical needs arose, and the members sat and read books to those who were in body casts and couldn't sit up. The Shriners also fell into step, hosting the children for special performances of the Shrine Circus and collecting gifts and clothes for holiday parties.

Although Junior Leaguer Justine Milam had young children at home, once a week she would hire a babysitter and volunteer at the Home. "I had my hands full with four little boys, but going to the Home renewed my vigor," she said. "I look back now and realize it probably saved my life."[31]

Some former patients, however, look back on their days at the Home with less-than-fond memories. "We were busy during the day, because we spent half the day in the classroom and the other half in physical or occupational therapy," Lancaster said. "They would prop pillows under my body cast so I could paint or crochet. But this was before television and [in the evenings] we children were left with nothing to do but look at the ceiling."[32]

Teenage boys and girls were kept separate during free periods. The League later built a long enclosed sunroom for the older patients, with a wide hall dividing the boys' side from the girls'. By pushing her body forward, Mary Ann Johns could scoot her bed forward just enough to see the boys' ward. She'd wave flirtatiously and the boys would wave back. "We were teenagers and we had the same hormones [as everybody else]," she said.[33]

Recalled Lancaster:

> We weren't allowed to mingle. One girl had juvenile arthritis and she was the only ambulatory person on the sun-porch, and she'd fetch and get for the rest of us. She was our go-between. Another girl was able to get up in a wheelchair and she'd sneak over to the boys' side at nighttime. One boy on crutches came over to our side after bed-check. The nurses checked our beds around ten or ten-thirty, and they didn't come back until five-thirty in the morning.

Maturity and hindsight often change one's view of a traumatic event. Lancaster admitted that part of her resentment towards the Home is tied up with her parents' divorce.

> My mother couldn't take care of me. My grandmother had had a stroke and so Mother was a single woman with two invalids on her hands. I was able to go home only one time. Mother hired an ambulance to bring me home for Easter. I was in an ambulance and a heavy body cast, and it was really traumatic as they tried to get me up the staircase.[34]

Former patient Helen Clark's memories mingle with gratitude. She explained:

> I must make testimony to the Junior League of Nashville, because at a time when women didn't go to Harvard Business School and there was no Vanderbilt School of Management or Business, the women who masterminded, conceptualized, worked their derrières off to put together the Junior League Home, to coordinate and pull in the Al Menah Temple Shriners, . . . I decided the women of the Junior League who were the leaders could . . . manage the State Department and the Department of the Army!

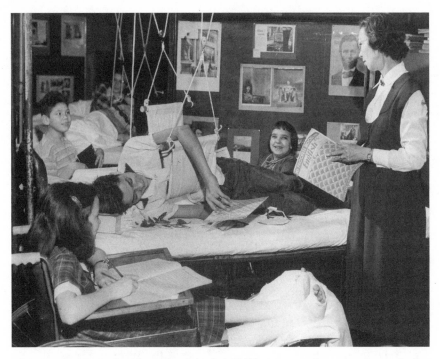

Boys and girls at the Home for Crippled Children were allowed to intermingle during meals and class time only.

"I mean," added Clark, raising her arm high for emphasis, "EXCELSIOR!"[35]

As far as Vanderbilt was concerned, the Junior League Home was a nice addition to the city, but the two institutions functioned as disparate solar systems whose orbits only occasionally and tangentially crossed. Many patients spent the early, acute stages of their illness as inpatients at Vanderbilt University Hospital before transferring to the Junior League Home to convalesce. Because Vanderbilt accepted charity cases, doctors in its clinics also handled these patients' non-orthopedic medical issues. Some Vanderbilt orthopedic surgeons gave diligent follow-up care to children at the Home, as did a few Vanderbilt pediatricians. However, most of the pediatricians who volunteered at the Home were local private practitioners, and quite a few of those were husbands of Junior League members.

By the early 1940s, the relationship between Vanderbilt and the Junior League had settled into a predictable arrangement, somewhat distant and exceedingly cordial. It would remain so until outside forces

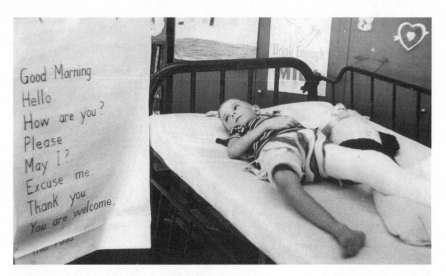

Proper manners and social skills were part of the curriculum at the Home.
Photo by J. F. Corn, Nashville Tennessean.

intervened and inside personalities clashed, slinging the two together and breaking the two apart, like ice floes riding on rough seas.

This all started with the death of one doctor and the arrival of another.

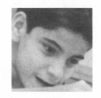

The Chief Arrives | 4

"In the [pediatrics] department there were two rules.
One of them was that if you have a teaching assignment,
you meet it or you get somebody to cover it.
Don't ask the secretaries. Don't ask [the Chairman].
You do it. But you never leave the students waiting.
Never. That was rule number one.
Rule number two was: No drinking at lunch."

—Dr. Robert Merrill, former medical student
and instructor under Dr. Amos Christie

In November 1942, World War II was going full throttle in the European, African, and Pacific theaters. On the eleventh day of that month, Adolph Hitler ordered the occupation of Vichy, France, and Allied troops attacked German forces in North Africa, leading to a stunning victory for General Dwight D. Eisenhower. On that same day, Dr. Horton Casparis died suddenly of a heart attack while attending the annual conference of the Southern Medical Association in Richmond, Virginia. With Casparis's untimely death at age fifty-one, Vanderbilt Hospital lost its chairman of pediatrics.

Having trained at Johns Hopkins Hospital, Casparis had arrived in Nashville in 1925, bringing with him his respected colleague Dr. Katherine Dodd. Earlier in his life, Casparis had spent a year in a sanitarium recovering from tuberculosis. The experience affected him profoundly and after he completed medical school, he channeled his research time into the study, treatment, and prevention of that disease, as well as other pediatric public health issues. He was a true public health clinician, focusing

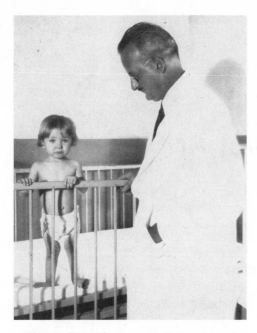

When Pediatric Chairman Dr. Horton Casparis died suddenly, the Vanderbilt administration had to find his replacement even though many faculty were off fighting in World War II.

on the welfare of the child—including nutrition, housing, education, child care, discipline, and mental and emotional status—as well as the disease or injury that led to a stay in the hospital.[1, 2]

As a junior pre-med student at Vanderbilt, Dr. William DeLoache attended Casparis's lectures, delivered with a cigarette dangling from his mouth, his stubby fingers stained with tobacco. "He'd say, 'Every child needs *security*,'" DeLoache recalled. "Now they call it self-esteem. This was his version of our current feeling that children should be assured of their self-worth. 'Security' was the buzzword of the time."

It's interesting that Casparis was so attuned to children's feelings, given the environment on the pediatric ward. Parents were not allowed to visit "unless the child was on death's door." "The head nurse on pediatrics was a tough old bird and I think nobody had the nerve to challenge the visitation policies she was so adamant about," DeLoache said. "She ruled the house staff pretty strictly, too. She believed that children were upset by parents visiting, because they cried when the parents left—and that could be avoided by not allowing parents to visit their children."

He added wryly, "I don't think Dr. Casparis's feelings about security were transposed onto the pediatric wards. They were primarily for the home."[3]

With Casparis's death, Vanderbilt administrators named Katherine Dodd to be the acting chair of pediatrics, the first female to hold such a position outside of nursing[4], while they formed a search committee to find a replacement for Casparis. This was no easy task. Medical faculties all across the United States foundered as young men went off to battle and returned home undereducated, distracted, or injured. Medical schools faced huge gaps in their internship, residency, and fellowship training programs. In addition to the depletion of younger house staff, half of Vanderbilt's senior medical staff left to fulfill military obligations. Somehow, Chancellor O. C. Carmichael and the Board of Trust had to unearth a middle-aged academic pediatric physician willing to relocate to a medical school that was long on potential but short on both personnel and financial support.

They discovered Dr. Amos Christie at the national offices of the American Red Cross.

Born in the timber camps of Eureka, California, Christie was the only child of a lumberjack who died at a young age, leaving an impoverished wife with a four-year-old son to raise. Amos and his mother lived in a room in the Union Labor Hospital, where Edna Christie worked as a cook/dietician and Amos grew up doing odd jobs and running errands to earn extra money.[5]

According to Christie, he and his mother were so busy working, clinging to the bond between them and trying not to disappoint each other, that they never had time to take stock of just how poor they were. "I think all she ever expected of me was not to get in jail," he wrote.[6]

At age sixteen, he tried to enlist in the navy to join the First World War, but Edna found out about it and dragged him home. The war ended with Amos "on top of a lumber pile at Armistice time" and still in high school.[7]

Having missed out on a naval career, Christie instead took to football, winning an athletic scholarship to the University of Washington and playing on a talented team that made it to two Rose Bowl championships. Although tall and muscular, Christie was usually relegated to second-string tackle for the Huskies. Occasionally, he was bumped up to first string. In later years, after he had earned a reputation as one of the world's leading clinical pediatricians, an aura of myth and legend evolved around this giant-sized man. At meetings and lectures he was introduced as a former All-American football star.[8]

To his credit, Christie never made that claim. On the other hand, his former protégé, Dr. Harris "Pete" Riley, remarked with a smile, "He did nothing to discourage it."[9]

In 1924, Christie entered the University of California Medical School at Berkeley, where he indulged in the rough nightlife of San Francisco's speakeasy saloons and still managed to make high enough grades to be accepted for a position at the Babies Hospital in New York City. To pay for the bicoastal trip, Christie took a job on a prison train, treating

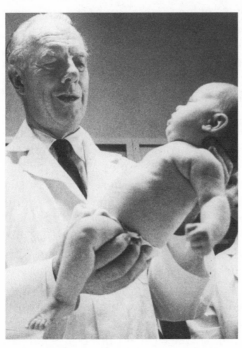

In 1943, Dr. Amos Christie became chairman of the Vanderbilt pediatrics department, a position he held for the next twenty-five years.

syphilis, tube feeding mental patients, and changing dirty wound dressings until he and the convicts disembarked on Ellis Island. A year later, he was back in the Bay Area as an instructor in the University of California's pediatric department. He then took a position at Johns Hopkins University on the Newborn Service, returned to California, and left again for the East Coast where he worked for the American Red Cross in Washington, D.C. It was here that the associate dean of Vanderbilt Medical School, renowned pathologist Dr. Ernest W. Goodpasture, found and recruited him.[10]

By this time, the Second World War was shifting course. The Red Cross blood plasma and collection program that had been so vital for the Allied forces was, of necessity, losing steam. Amos Christie needed a new challenge, and he desperately wanted to teach. Chancellor Carmichael sent Christie an official letter on July 24, 1943, asking him to become professor and chairman of pediatrics at Vanderbilt for an annual salary of eight thousand dollars, with potential private practice privileges of two hundred dollars annually, and a moving allowance of six hundred dollars.[11] Only someone working for the federal government would have considered that a generous offer. Christie took the job.

Back in Nashville, Dr. Katie Dodd was not pleased. She was, by all rights, the logical person to be named head of the department. She was a popular teacher, respected scientist, and devoted and aggressive clinician who arrived an hour early every morning to check on all the patients *before* the residents came in to give rounds.[12] In other words, she essentially rounded twice each morning. To be replaced by a man who had not even been practicing pediatrics for the past few years—much less someone unknown in scholarly circles—did not sit well with her.[13] In truth, Dodd likely never had a chance. Naming a woman as chair of a major medical department was simply too radical a concept for Vanderbilt in the 1940s.

Christie let Dodd know exactly where he stood. He wrote in his memoir:

> I explained . . . I had had a long record of being able to get along well with women in medicine. I expected them to conduct themselves like other colleagues and not ask for special privileges because they were women, but rather to hold their end up in every way. I was sure Dr. Dodd would do this, at the same time making it clear that I was going to be the Chairman of the Department.
> She accepted this, in retrospect, somewhat reluctantly.[14]

In fact, she soon moved to Cincinnati and took a job at the Children's Hospital in that city. Years later, Dodd was named chairman of pediatrics at the University of Arkansas.[15]

Christie's relationship with female faculty members was always, at best, colorful. As part of his new Vanderbilt faculty, he had inherited Dr. Ann Minot, a PhD and a well-liked associate professor of pediatric research. "It happened that I needed a Research Associate of Pediatrics during this transitional period in the department like I needed another hole in my head," Christie wrote.[16]

Minot subsequently moved to the Department of Biochemistry.

Yet there were two women in the pediatrics department that Christie could never shake loose. They would stand their ground for decades, forging inroads into medical science sometimes because of and sometimes despite their Chairman. One was Dr. Mildred Stahlman and the other was Dr. Sarah Sell. Their academic contributions, among others in the department, would ultimately put Vanderbilt pediatrics on a fast-moving train that even Amos Christie could not stop.

Mildred Stahlman was in Christie's first medical school class. A petite, pretty young woman with dark hair piled atop her head, she was the youngest daughter of James Stahlman, the controversial publisher of the *Nashville Banner*. Like her father, Millie was a force to be reckoned with. Born into privilege, she attended Nashville's prestigious Ward-Belmont finishing school for young ladies. Encouraged by her father to be tough-minded and independent, she decided as a child that she would grow up to be a doctor, an unusual choice of profession for a high-born Southern girl. When she entered Vanderbilt Medical School in 1943, she was one of four women in a class of fifty.[17]

By the time she received her MD degree, Stahlman was at a crossroads. She wanted to subspecialize and Amos Christie didn't believe in subspecialization. Every decent pediatrician, he swore, needed to be a generalist. They must understand equally the heart, lungs, gastrointestinal tract, ears, nose, and throat. They should be capable of making physical diagnoses, stitching up wounds, drawing blood gases, and reading X-rays. How else could they properly take care of children? Research, however, was moving in the direction of tighter and tighter focus on particular physiological systems and a more specialized division of labor. Many young doctors, including Stahlman, were following the rising tide.

While attending a fellowship program at the famed Karolinska Institute in Stockholm, Sweden, Stahlman became hooked on the care of newborn infants. She also began to see the world from a more liberal standpoint than upscale Nashville society, or her own upbringing, had offered. The welfare of children, she came to believe, was as much a political as a cultural responsibility.[18]

Back at Vanderbilt, she returned not to pediatrics, but to the physiology department, where she worked for seven years under Dr. Elliott V. Newman, founder of Vanderbilt's Clinical Research Center. Stahlman directed her research efforts toward solving pediatric cardiopulmonary problems.[19]

When Christie found out she would be training under Newman, he tried to talk her out of it. "You'll be back," he told her. "Your place is at the bedside."

"Sure, I did come back," she said later, "but I came back with a totally different set of skills—what I'd learned in seven years of residency training. I was prepared to run a research unit, and to not just take care of patients."[20]

Unforeseen by Christie, Stahlman rejoined the pediatrics faculty with more spit-and-vinegar and creative resolve than ever, ultimately becoming one of the early pioneers in the new field of neonatology. Many times, she would be almost more than her chairman could handle.

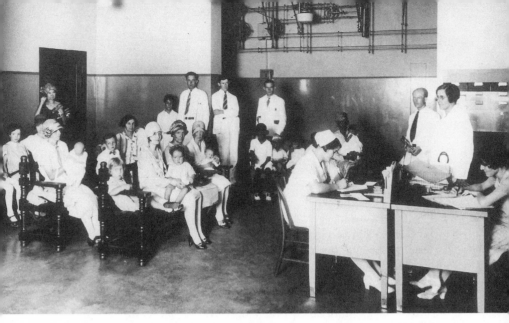

Even by the standards of the day, the pediatric clinic at Vanderbilt, here run by Dr. Katie Dodd (standing right), was considered bare-boned and austere.

When Sarah Sell began her first year of medical school, she already had a world of experience behind her. She was married to a young doctor, had a master's degree in microbiology, and had spent the past six years working for a federal welfare program in rural West Virginia, delivering health care to indigent people in the Appalachian Mountains. Trained as a basic scientist, but finding herself far removed from the laboratory bench, Sell read manuals on gardening and midwifery and, side by side with her husband, embarked on a life of idealistic social service. In 1941, she and her husband made a temporary move to Nashville so he could receive further training at St. Thomas Hospital in surgery, which he felt he needed for his rural general practice. When the United States joined the war, he volunteered to go overseas, as did many of his colleagues.

Before he shipped out, however, he went to Vanderbilt and petitioned the admissions committee to offer his wife a spot in the medical school. He believed that if Sarah earned her MD degree, they could provide an even better service to the poor folks in West Virginia after he returned from his tour of duty. At that time, hundreds of young service men were attending medical school programs as part of their army or navy assignments, so he knew that getting his wife into medical school was a long shot. Still, Vanderbilt had one opening and Goodpasture offered it to Sarah. She was one of two women admitted that year. The other woman dropped out after a month.

Sell recalled:

> We were first assigned to Anatomy. There was a black man named Bill who helped the students with odds and ends in anatomy. Bill was a great guy. He had seen many, many medical students. We had groups of four on a cadaver and three navy boys invited me to fill out their fourth position. Bill came up and said, "You boys are lucky to have a lady with you, and Dr. Sam Clark, who's head of this course in anatomy, he's a gentleman. Dr. Sam Clark is a gentle person and he is very quiet. But if you are unkind to this lady, he's a lion. He'll come in and roar at you. So you be kind to this lady and you help her." [21]

Those boys paid attention. Anatomy, in those days, was not so much taught as directed. The students were given a *Gray's Anatomy* textbook and a course outline and were left to figure out the intimacies of the human body on their own. On their first day of class, they were essentially provided this much instruction: "Start on the leg."[22]

Dr. Amos Christie (front row, third from left) wanted to keep his department small and excellent. Dr. Mildred Stahlman is front row, second from left. Dr. Sarah Sell is front row, second from right.

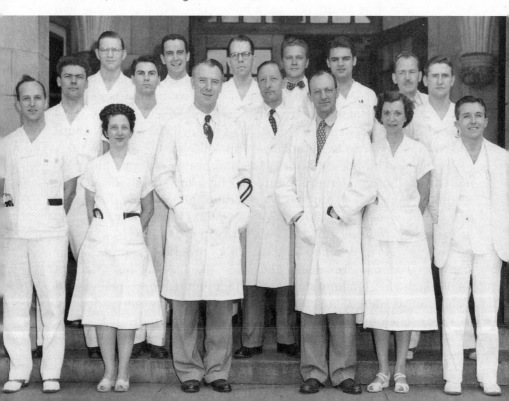

With two people on each side, one student read out the instructions, another read from the anatomy text, trying to decipher the foreign Greek- and Latin-based medical terms, while the other two students took turns dissecting the cadaver. A professor appeared at the end of the week to check off and grade them on what they'd accomplished.[23]

During Sell's sophomore year, her husband was killed in the war. With nowhere else to go, she stayed in medical school and graduated in 1948. Over the course of her career, she would remarry and have children, join the pediatrics faculty as an expert in infectious disease, become the first woman to serve as president of the Nashville Academy of Medicine, and be instrumental in the development of childhood vaccines, including one that protects against the killer *Haemophilus influenzae* type B (HIB) virus.

All of which is to say that when Amos Christie became chairman of pediatrics at Vanderbilt Medical School, he was innocently stepping into a cauldron of contradictory dynamics. Medical residents were being called off to war. Female medical students were setting their sights not simply on general practice, but on careers as academicians. New technological interventions, spawned by the war effort, were being applied to the treatment of sick children. In the laboratory, scientists were working on future blockbuster drugs like penicillin that would shortly begin altering the standard of patient care.

Medical historian and ethicist Dr. Stuart Finder explains the changes this way: Although medicine had been evolving throughout the late nineteenth century, it was really during and after World War II that the government began routing a "radical infusion of cash" into universities for research into new technologies—both drug technologies and surgical devices. Each year, on each front, new things began coming out of scientific medicine that transformed the practice of medicine.[24]

Finder said, "So, a tension starts to develop between the mission for care, the mission for research and the mission for education. Vanderbilt begins trying to establish itself in this research paradigm, because that's how medicine as a whole is going. That's where the power is. That's where the money is."[25] In fact, between 1925 and 1935, Vanderbilt medical researchers had already launched several major discoveries.[26]

In the midst of this swelling tension stood Amos Christie, who considered his primary mission to be education. Never one to equivocate, he believed that if his students and residents acquired

the best training, then it would naturally follow that patients on his
ward would receive outstanding care. He was also certain that residents had to first become competent health care providers and had
to first understand illnesses in children if their research interests
were to have translational value.

His own research was a case in point. Children all over the central
and eastern United States were believed to have tuberculosis because
they had spots on the lung that appeared as calcifications on X-ray.
Having had prior experience with a fungal infection among children
in California, Christie suspected something else was at play, and he
conducted a series of experiments to find out.

Every child who entered Vanderbilt Hospital—whether it was for
a hernia repair, tonsillectomy, or a major illness—was given a skin test
for tuberculosis and also for histoplasmosis, a lung disease caused by a
fungus that grows in soil and other material contaminated with bat or
bird droppings. Along with Dr. J. C. Peterson, Christie showed that the
vast majority of children in his study tested positive for histoplasmosis,
and very few actually had tuberculosis.[27] Fortunately, unlike tuberculosis, histoplasmosis could not be passed from person to person. This
and later clinical research, which was relatively straightforward and
uncomplicated, earned him great acclaim and numerous awards as the
world's leading expert on that disease. He'd honed his expertise in
histoplasmosis by acquiring knowledge about a variety of disease
processes in children and applying that knowledge to real-life cases.
Confident that his was the best approach to medical research, he felt
compelled to pass it along to upcoming generations of pediatricians.

With such an impassioned conviction about the value of teaching,
Christie, who had joined the Vanderbilt faculty as a distinct outsider,
quickly engendered loyalty and love from his medical students and
residents. The Vanderbilt pediatric program became renowned not
only within the institution, but nationwide, for its excellence, its inten-
sity, and its freewheeling approach to the training of young doctors.[28]
In other words, the house staff under Amos Christie operated on a
system of implied, rather than stated parameters. His minions shared
one major goal—not to let the Chief down.

Said Dr. Robert Merrill, one of Christie's former medical
students, who later joined the faculty as an instructor, "In the [pedi-
atrics] department there were two rules. One of them was that if you
have a teaching assignment, you meet it or you get somebody to
cover it. Don't ask the secretaries. Don't ask [the Chairman]. You do

it. But you never leave the students waiting. Never. That was rule number one.

"Rule number two was: No drinking at lunch."[29]

Merrill added that, in reality, the house staff operated under a tight system of unstated guidelines about responsibility, thoroughness, and knowledge about patients. For example, if a resident ordered an X-ray on a patient, he was expected to go to the radiology department and read the X-ray himself. "If you didn't go to look at it, then it wasn't worth ordering," Merrill said. "That discipline was all unwritten, but it was there."[30]

If members of the house staff fell short, Christie never berated or chastised them, but he let them know his opinion. For example, if a patient was admitted late at night, the resident was expected to perform the appropriate lab work. If the resident left out a certain test that should have been run, Christie would simply comment on rounds the next morning, "Next time you're in a vein, draw serum calciums."

"We had to explain to new residents that what that meant was, 'Why in the hell didn't you get a serum calcium?'" Merrill said.[31]

Dr. William Altemeier recalls a similar incident during his residency. A fourteen-year-old girl with severe lupus was admitted to the hospital. Hydrocortisone had just been introduced as a treatment for lupus, but as a new drug, it had both known and unknown side effects. On rounds, the residents asked whether they could treat her with hydrocortisone, and Christie responded that he thought that would be a bad idea. "Don't do it," he said. End of story.

Except Altemeier and his fellow resident on call decided to give it a try. A day and a half later, the patient developed an acute psychotic break (which, in hindsight, may not have been from the lupus or the drug) and began yelling, screaming, and thrashing around. The panicked residents moved her down the hall, tried to put her in isolation, and keep her as quiet as possible—and they also prevented Christie from seeing her. A few days later she came out of her psychosis, and with a sigh of relief, the residents discharged her from the hospital. No harm done.

Months later, Altemeier was speaking to Christie and that particular case came up. "Oh," said Altemeier, "do you remember that patient?"

"Yes," Christie harumphed. "I told you not to give her steroids!" He'd known the whole time what had gone on, had made sure the patient wouldn't suffer any long-term damage, and had never said a word to his residents.

Altemeier explained, "It was a resident-centered teaching program. We not only had the authority to manage the patients, we had the responsibility. That's a way to really grow up. That makes good doctors."

"It would be illegal today," he added.[32]

Christie had so much confidence in his residents' ability to run the service that he allowed them to police themselves when he was out of town for a day or two. Protocol dictated otherwise. On the unit was a chalkboard where he was supposed to write the name of the person appointed to be the acting chief during his absence. Under acting chairman, Christie was known to inscribe "Jack Daniel."[33]

In this atmosphere and era, young pediatricians thrived. They understood the chain of command—if they hustled, studied, and demonstrated loyalty, then they would be protected. They knew that if they got into trouble—which happens regularly in a high-tension, crisis-centered medical institute—they were obliged to let their Chairman know immediately.

One night Bob Merrill was serving as the admitting officer on a busy night at Vanderbilt Hospital. It was late, he was exhausted, and the admissions office took issue with a patient that Merrill had admitted. Merrill and the staff member got into an argument that devolved into a heated exchange with the hospital administrator. Finally, the young resident lost his composure and said some things he quickly regretted. In an instant, he bounded up the three flights of stairs to his Chairman's office, only to find Christie already on the phone.

"He said what? He did what? Really?" an incredulous Christie asked. "Well, I'm sorry that happened. I'm really sorry, but he was *right*. He was absolutely right and he did absolutely the right thing. Yes, we can talk about this later."

Christie put the phone down, looked up at Merrill, and said, "Don't you EVER do that again!"

Deeply indebted, Merrill fled the office.[34]

In another instance, a frustrated resident once became so riled by an X-ray technician that he cold-cocked the guy—knocked him flat. Christie came into his office early the next morning to find the resident already standing there, ready to explain what had happened. The chairman immediately sent him on vacation. Later that morning, an irate hospital administrator arrived at his door to complain about the behavior of his resident. "That's terrible!" Christie said, feigning surprise. "But the young man is on vacation this week. Don't worry. I will speak to him about this as soon as he returns."

Said one former resident, "You would walk through fire for a guy like that!"[35]

Faculty and house staff found it thrilling to be part of the team. In those days, the medical and university faculty ate lunch together in the same cafeteria. Biologists and physicians discussed ideas of mutual interest. Colleagues from medicine, pathology, and surgery shared thoughts over hamburgers and french fries. Instructors or adjunct professors would seek out veteran faculty members working in their laboratories and ask them for a consult on a particular patient. Together they'd go to the patient's room and try to figure out problems. Nobody billed for time spent on a consult. Nobody worried about ruffling feathers.[36]

"The cross-fertilization was magnificent. It was just a marvelous environment," Merrill said.

They were a fraternity—with a few sorority sisters among their ranks. And, like a fraternal enclave of the elite, the handpicked protégés of Amos Christie developed an air of cockiness nurtured within an insulated shell. "Let's keep it small and let's keep it good," became the pediatric department's motto.[37]

During the post–World War II era, doctors were becoming increasingly respected within their communities, but were rarely financially enriched by their profession. Even the most active pediatrician in private practice was a solid middle-class citizen. On the other hand, academic physicians were often, at best, eking by on blue-collar wages, particularly at small Southern medical centers like Vanderbilt. In the case of Christie's group, the lack of funds tended to unite his faculty. They knew their Chief's salary, like theirs, was barely subsistence level. They bonded in poverty. For them, the practice of medicine was a calling rather than a career. Wives and husbands from Vanderbilt became the "ins." Everybody else was considered an outsider.

Recalled Bennie Batson, whose husband, Randy, became Christie's right-hand man on faculty, "People were extremely close. The heads of departments and instructors—all the staff were buddies. They went fishing together. They hunted together. They socialized. That was my life. I saw very little of town people. It was a problem. It boiled down to hate. A lot of the town people hated Vanderbilt."[38]

It was actually closer to love-hate. Vanderbilt physicians often referred to their patients as "teaching material," and even those children from families capable of paying were treated as charity cases. Yet, around Nashville, Christie also became revered as a savior of young lives. Families shared stories of his rescuing a child who was choking to death; of his correctly diagnosing an obscure, but treatable, disease in a suffering youngster; or of his lifting a tiny infant into his massive hands and quieting the colicky baby. In essence, Nashvillians simultaneously admired and resented those renegade Vanderbilt doctors, and only ventured into the teaching hospital if they were so poor or if a child was in such dire straits that they had no other choice.

Such a relationship suited Amos Christie just fine. He was more than happy to avoid scrutiny by the local citizenry. He was an avid outdoorsman and liked nothing better than taking a colleague or a junior faculty member and a flask of whiskey down the Buffalo River for a leisurely weekend fishing expedition.[39] He told his residents, "If you're too busy to go fishing, you're too busy." He expected his people to take time off when they needed it.[40]

Every year, Christie and his wife, Margaret, threw parties for the incoming house staff. Margaret was a beautiful woman with a lovely figure and a flamboyant personality. When Christie met her, she was an actress who'd been cast as an understudy to Jeannette McDonald. After moving to Nashville, she was generally relegated to roles in local community theater. The parties at the Christie home were legendary. After a few rounds of beer, Margaret would shuffle everybody aside to play show tunes on the piano, and the guests would join in a raucous sing-along.

Christie would also organize periodic road trips to college football games. On one such trip, his busload of revelers arrived in Memphis at the Peabody Hotel, only to find that there had been some miscommunication and all the rooms were full. To accommodate the tired swarm of late arrivals and with nowhere else to put them, the hotel personnel allowed the Vanderbilt crowd to sleep in meeting rooms and broom closets.

"It was fun," Bennie Batson said. "And we all forgave Dr. Christie."[41]

Another annual event was the departmental party at the Jack Daniel Distillery in Lynchburg, Tennessee. The Motlow family owned the distillery and had made generous contributions to the Vanderbilt pediatric department. To celebrate, Christie would charter a bus, and leaving a skeleton crew behind to care for the inpatients, load up all the interns, residents, wives, and faculty for a big hoedown barbecue.

They would tour the distillery, which was—and still is—in a dry county. Undeterred, they'd then load up the bus and drive to the next county, which was wet, sample the whiskey, and dance to fiddle music. Armed with a survival kit for the ride home, they'd return to Nashville singing obscene songs and making up obscene limericks.

"The relationship between the department and the distillery was quite intimate," quipped Bob Merrill.[42]

If the Vanderbilt pediatric unit seemed to be one big party, it was far from that. Christie may have been given free rein to educate his young house staff as he saw fit, but he could not dictate the mores of the institution. In the early 1940s, black patients could be admitted to Vanderbilt Hospital, but both children and adults were kept together on a separate unit known as 8400, "the Negro ward." At that time departmental chairmen were practically omnipotent and they had final say whether or not their staff would take care of minority patients. For the most part, pediatric faculty did and surgery faculty did not.

Amos Christie was not raised in the South and he found racial segregation perplexing and counterproductive, particularly at a teaching hospital that catered to charity patients. The problems inherent on 8400 gnawed at him for years. When his daughter and only child Linda was a preschooler, she was hospitalized for a tonsillectomy operation on Vanderbilt's pediatric unit. Her father walked into her room, deeply troubled. "This looks so much better than the Negro ward does, and I don't like the difference," Christie said to her. "There should be no differences for children."[43]

A few years after that, Christie, in his inimitable style, addressed the problem. Exactly what happened continues to be debated, and Christie himself told different versions of the story in his memoir and in various letters. As best as can be determined, the impetus once again boiled down to the teaching program. Sometime between 1946 and 1948, long before *Brown v. the Board of Education* or other mandatory racial integration laws, a white child was hospitalized with chicken pox on the pediatric unit, Ward 4300, and kept in an isolated room because of the contagiousness of the illness. At the same time, on 8400, a black child was also hospitalized with chicken pox. The resident taking care of both children was running himself ragged going from end to end of the hospital tending to each child.

Christie had had enough. One night he and Randy Batson simply walked into the black child's room, unlocked the bed, and pushed it down to the pediatric unit and into the room of the white patient. Now the resident could deliver care to both children more easily.[44]

Recalled Bob Merrill, "Dr. Christie said, '*This* is where we're going to take care of black babies . . . If we're going to take care of babies, we're going to take care of them correctly.' End of discussion. He didn't ask anybody. He didn't get a committee going. The dean didn't know it. The hospital administration didn't know it. He just did it. His attitude was, if you don't like it, come see me."[45]

Remarkably, Christie suffered little, if any, repercussions from his bold decision. He had figured out that despite all the prescient hand-waving, it was actually much easier to desegregate than to resegregate. Once word got out, however, white townspeople became that much more wary of Vanderbilt. They knew that if their own sick children had to be admitted to that hospital, they might easily room with black children. Many Nashvillians were not prepared for that.

In his memoir, Christie justified his decision to integrate for financial reasons. Vanderbilt, he wrote, began to get into financial difficulty in the late 1940s and as part of the solution to the problem, Dean Goodpasture and Mr. Clarence Connell, director of the Hospital, decided to shut down the Negro ward, including its six pediatric beds, so that private, paying white patients could have those rooms instead. Christie was not willing to give up those pediatric beds, and hence, transferred them to Ward 4300.

Christie writes:

> There were many dividends from this move. The teaching service could have more material, particularly as the Negro community became more affluent and was covered by Blue Cross-Blue Shield insurance. You always benefit by doing the right thing. I learned a lot about race and human relations as Pediatrics led the pack again. I was additionally rewarded by an invitation to address the John Andrews Clinical Society in Tuskegee [Alabama] in 1955. I interpreted this as recognition of my efforts toward improvement of race relations.[46]

Race relations aside, by the time Christie integrated the pediatric ward, Vanderbilt Hospital and Vanderbilt Medical School, like many teaching hospitals recovering from World War II, had been beating back financial crises for a number of years. The lack of institutional money and the mismanagement of billing services would ultimately incite a ferocious battle between the medical administration, the Board of Trust, and the medical faculty. The rifts and wounds created by that conflict would fester for many years, leaving behind a distaste for financial risk and an aversion toward building a children's hospital.

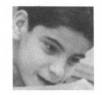

On the Brink of
Financial Catastrophe | 5

Merrill: *"May I see private patients?"*

Christie: *"Well, yeah, if you want to."*

Merrill: *"Which ones should I see?"*

Christie: *"Whichever ones come along—if you want to."*

Merrill: *"Should I bill them?"*

Christie: *"Well, yeah."*

Merrill: *"Do we have a fee schedule?"*

Christie: *"No, I don't think we do."*

Merrill: *"Well, how much should I charge?"*

Christie: *"Whatever you think is appropriate."*

**—Dr. Robert Merrill, relating a conversation
with Pediatrics Chairman Amos Christie,
after Merrill joined the faculty as an instructor**

By the middle of the twentieth century, Vanderbilt's determination to be above and apart from the surrounding community almost brought the Medical Center to its knees. Like Cassandra calling to the Trojans, Dean Goodpasture had been warning his colleagues for a long time that a crisis was brewing. Vanderbilt faced a pair of intractable dilemmas: One, its hospital was on the verge of bankruptcy; two, so was its medical school.

Dr. Ernest Goodpasture had come to Vanderbilt in 1925 as the chairman of pathology. He was a bred-in-the-bone basic scientist, and

53

a brilliant one at that. By the time he assumed the position of dean in 1945, he had already received international acclaim for his work on mumps, fowlpox, and vaccinia (a viral relative of smallpox), and had developed a breakthrough technique for growing viruses in chicken embryos. The chick embryo technique, which he gave to Upjohn Pharmaceuticals free of charge and with no strings attached, meant that drug companies could begin producing mass quantities of vaccines against yellow fever, typhus, influenza, and Rocky Mountain Spotted Fever. Goodpasture's unselfish act and willingness to share scientific knowledge would ultimately save millions of lives around the world.[1]

If Vanderbilt, meanwhile, aspired to establish itself as a serious player in the world of academics, and if it were going to compete for power and prestige against Harvard, Duke, and Columbia, it would have to invest heavily in faculty research. In the mid-twentieth century, medical research was experiencing an explosion, and it, rather than patient care or superb teaching, was the sphere that was putting medical institutions on the map—a place where Vanderbilt eagerly wanted to be.[2]

Unfortunately, America was also entering a period of postwar inflation, which made advanced medical services all the more costly. Vanderbilt's nursing staff and support staff of housekeepers and laboratory technicians were grossly underpaid and were often quick to depart for more lucrative jobs elsewhere. Without nurses to staff the beds, doctors had to keep the hospital census low, hovering around a dismal 65 percent of capacity. The physical plant had deteriorated and was in desperate need of major repairs. In 1945, Chancellor Oliver C. Carmichael, who had replaced Kirkland eight years earlier, resigned to become head of the Carnegie Foundation. So Vanderbilt decision-makers simultaneously faced a fiscal crisis and a lame-duck administration. And finally, the medical school and hospital were both limping along with an underfunded endowment and "an archaic accounting system" for processing income.[3]

As a result, in the mid-1940s, Vanderbilt Hospital ended each year with a chronic, substantial deficit, forcing administrators to dip into a dwindling reserve fund. The School of Medicine (which was under Dean Goodpasture's aegis—the hospital was not) fared a little better. Still, the combined deficits of the two enterprises for the three-year period between 1946–48 rose to over $400,000, with a meager $46,500 remaining in reserves.[4]

Explained Dr. Henry Clark, who was appointed hospital director in 1948:

> . . . there had developed a general feeling of hopelessness among the once proud professional and lay staff of the hospital . . . More important, there seemed to be no prospects of new money, with the result that salaries of all faculty members were frozen . . . Even more important, the scientific world was burgeoning in the wake of World War II and it was impossible to appoint new personnel to stay abreast of the times . . .[5]

Into this conundrum waltzed a new Chancellor, Harvie Branscomb. Born in Birmingham, Alabama, and a graduate of Birmingham Southern University, Branscomb was both a theologian and a son of the Deep South. He wanted Vanderbilt to become a leading national university, and he knew that the hospital and medical school would have to remain solvent for that to happen. This was no time for excuses; Dean Goodpasture and hospital director C. P. Connell had to fix the problem.

The dean and the hospital director first tried a number of belt-tightening moves to remedy the situation. They began charging indigent patients a flat rate of $8.50 a day for hospitalization. They solicited local businessmen and established what became known as "The Desperation Fund" to cover expenditures restricted to the purchase of expensive drugs, such as penicillin, which the hospital was unable to furnish to charity patients.[6] They told the faculty that, beginning

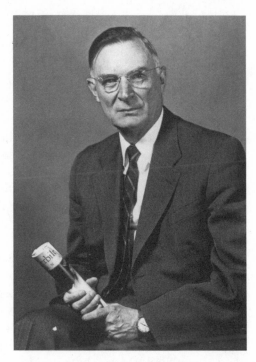

Dr. Harvie Branscomb served as Chancellor of Vanderbilt University during some of its most tumultuous times.

June 1, 1948, Ward 8400 would be closed as a Negro floor and opened instead to white private patients, although Vanderbilt would continue to admit "colored people" to the outpatient clinic. Finally, Goodpasture appointed a committee to evaluate four options: 1) balancing the medical school budget; 2) opening up the clinics to private practitioners; 3) leasing the hospital to the community; or 4) discontinuing the four-year medical school curriculum.[7] He appointed Amos Christie to head up that committee.

In the process of trying to salvage Vanderbilt's medical arm from bankruptcy, the Christie Committee (as it came to be called) was awakened to a harsh dose of reality. For one thing, Nashvillians as a whole could have cared less that their city's teaching hospital might go under. For over forty years, the mid-town hospital had been taking care of the indigent populace of Middle Tennessee. In exchange for these teaching opportunities, Vanderbilt had been operating without much financial backing or input from its surrounding citizenry. In his final report, dated December 30, 1948, Christie stated in a rather startled and hurt tone, "It may be doubted if any other institution in the country has been so lacking in local support and appreciation."[8]

Chancellor Branscomb agreed and went to the city managers, hat in hand, seeking financial assistance, lest they lose a fine teaching institution forever. According to historian Paul Conkin, "Branscomb believed Nashville did not deserve the school if it refused to help."[9] He proposed that Vanderbilt and Meharry take over the care of the city's black and/or indigent patients, who were currently being admitted to the dilapidated Nashville General Hospital. Vanderbilt asked the city to pay it a fee for each impoverished inpatient and outpatient seen by their doctors, and in exchange, it would add additional beds to care for Nashville's poorest citizens. If the city rejected the proposal, Branscomb insisted, Vanderbilt would no longer accept nonpaying indigent patients.

The situation evolved into a daring, toe-to-toe power play. Nashville rejected Branscomb's contract—and the Chancellor followed through on his threat. The hospital no longer provided free services, except in cases of emergency. Nashville's indigent population, pawns in the dispute, suddenly couldn't access health care anywhere.

The city backed down first. In 1949, city managers entered into a contract with both Vanderbilt and Meharry, with most black inpatients assigned to be cared for at Meharry and with Vanderbilt personnel staffing General Hospital.[10]

In the meantime, the Christie Committee was engaged in its own showdown. All across the country, medical research centers were finding, like Vanderbilt, that money was too scarce to support both a first-class research program and a superlative medical school. Amos Christie's lifeblood was the teaching program. He had no choice but to rescue it from the rubble.

"If research is allowed to die, education will remain static," he wrote in his report, "but if education dies there will be no research workers and ultimately both education and research will die. For this reason, the committee feels that at the moment the main emphasis should be the survival of the medical school."[11]

For a scientist like Dean Goodpasture, it was one thing to campaign for the medical school's survival but quite another to come

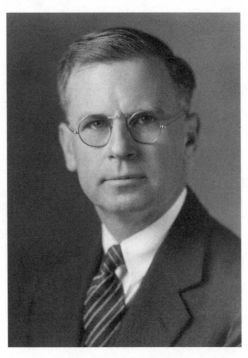

In the wake of a seemingly insurmountable post-war deficit, Dr. Ernest Goodpasture proposed that Vanderbilt close down its medical school and become a research institute.

up with quick, workable remedies to make that possible. He decided to play hardball. On January 7, 1949, he sent Branscomb a radical proposal: close Vanderbilt's four-year medical school and convert the facility into a research institute. He suggested the Chancellor discontinue at the earliest possible date the undergraduate curriculum of the medical school. In its stead, Vanderbilt should house an academy that was purely devoted to medical research and education at a graduate and postgraduate level.[12]

If Goodpasture's plan to eliminate premedical education was carried out, Vanderbilt Hospital would no longer function as a center for teaching interns and residents. Graduate and postgraduate students would work in laboratories alongside biomedical faculty to

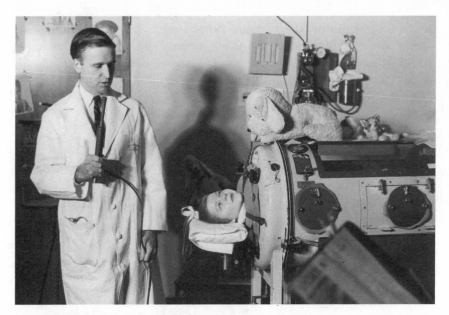

Dr. Robert Merrill taught medical students and residents about the care of patients in iron lung respirators.

receive their master's and PhD degrees, but no MD degrees would be conferred.[13] Goodpasture suggested that other local hospitals— Meharry, Nashville General, and the Veteran's Hospital—could assume the responsibility for providing "teaching material" and for training house staff.

A month later, the Board of Trust took Goodpasture's proposal under consideration and chose not to accept it. Although offering little in the way of hard solutions, the Christie Committee had won out. Frustrated that Vanderbilt was still struggling financially a year later, Goodpasture resigned over the imbroglio and returned full-time to his research endeavors. Said Dr. Robert Collins, author of the biography, *Ernest William Goodpasture: Scientist, Scholar, Gentleman*, "[Dr. Goodpasture] was a very principled person . . . and simply acted on his convictions."

By the early 1950s, Vanderbilt Hospital and Medical School would laboriously climb out of their fiscal catatonia—only to fall back time and again over the next thirty years.

By rejecting Goodpasture's proposal, Chancellor Branscomb was effectively sticking by his pediatric department chairman. Together they would ride out Vanderbilt's monetary disasters, buoyed by a confidence—perhaps overly optimistic, but a driving force all the same—in its potential to grow as an eminent center of learning. Years later, when Branscomb faced a new crisis within the university, Amos Christie would repay the favor.

It's ironic that Christie was named to head a committee on fiscal responsibility. He had joined the Vanderbilt faculty only two years earlier, and he was notorious for being a poor manager of money, both at home and at work. Money was often a sore subject with his family. "Well, I wish he could have balanced his checkbook," sighed his daughter Linda.

Pete Riley recalled, "We learned never to go behind him in the cafeteria line, because he never had any money. He'd have to borrow twenty-nine cents. Or he'd say he lost his checkbook."

In fact, Christie found the business side of his job to be singularly annoying. He viewed the practice of medicine as similar to missionary work, and charging people for medical expertise was almost hypocritical. Robert Merrill had been out in private practice when Christie asked him to return to Vanderbilt to be on the pediatrics faculty. Merrill took a pay cut in order to rejoin his mentor, agreeing to work for seventy-five-hundred dollars a year. With a bit of real-world experience under his belt, Merrill knew that some patients' families should be expected to pay for services rendered, but he didn't know the departmental rules. So he had a quick conversation with Christie:

> Merrill: "May I see private patients?"
> Christie: "Well, yeah, if you want to."
> Merrill: "Which ones should I see?"
> Christie: "Whichever ones come along—if you want to."
> Merrill: "Should I bill them?"
> Christie: "Well, yeah."
> Merrill: "Do we have a fee schedule?"
> Christie: "No, I don't think we do."
> Merrill: "Well, how much should I charge?"
> Christie: "Whatever you think is appropriate."
> Merrill: "What do I do with the bills?"
> Christie: "Give them to Anne [Hudgens, his assistant]."
> Merrill: "How will I know whether it's collected or not?"
> Christie: "She'll take care of it. Don't worry about it."[14]

"Can you imagine a more wonderful way to practice medicine?" Merrill exclaimed.

The department's collections, when received, were pooled into a general fund to cover books, meeting fees, and travel expenses. Merrill recalled one patient who had leukemia. The child's disease was exhausting the family's limited resources. On his own, Merrill quit turning in bills for that patient. His chairman never mentioned it. Christie's perspective, he said, was that if people didn't have the money, it wasn't appropriate to bill them. But if they did have money, it was all right to submit a bill. "He wasn't against [billing for services], he was just selective," said Merrill.[15]

Such an altruistic attitude—while a boon for patients and for a zealous faculty and house staff—did nothing to keep the institution afloat.

In its final report, the Christie Committee had set forth nine recommendations for improving the financial health of the institution. Recommendation number eight addressed an increasingly turbulent issue: "That those members of 'full-time' staff who are engaged in private practice be required to pay office rent and that other similar measures be sought to eliminate the criticism of 'unfair competition.'"[16] In other words, Christie wanted private doctors to shell out some cash for the privilege of working at Vanderbilt.

In truth, the role of private practitioners working at Vanderbilt Hospital had become touchy for both sides. Pediatrics was the perfect case in point. The idea of private doctors bossing around his residents and interfering with the care of his patients didn't sit well with Amos Christie. As a result, he was extremely selective in whom he would grant admitting privileges. Ironically, the majority of Nashville's pediatricians had graduated from Vanderbilt Medical School, and they did not appreciate being denied the right to admit there once they'd hung out their shingles. Now practicing in Nashville, they were suddenly cut off from the same hospitalized children they'd been slavishly tending to for years as residents.

"We didn't give them access lightly," Sarah Sell said. "Those whom Dr. Christie put on his faculty, he made them pay dearly to get in. They had to work in the clinic with the residents and do a lot of dirty work before he'd give them an appointment."[17]

In other words, town doctors had to agree to work at least one half-day a week at Vanderbilt's pediatric clinic if they wanted to join Christie's tribe. Plus, they had to be board-certified in pediatrics. Those who weren't board-certified were immediately eliminated from consideration. Also, Christie had to deem them qualified physicians before he'd open his door to them. He wanted the best physicians attending in his hospital. Needless to say, this created quite a riff among the "ins" and the "outs."

Dr. Eric Chazen, who did have admitting privileges, explained that doctors who hadn't made the cut but who had a sick child needing to come to Vanderbilt would have to admit their patients to a doctor on faculty. They didn't admit to a fellow private practitioner who might have privileges, because that would indicate to patients that their doctor hadn't made the grade. "To avoid that," Chazen said, "the 'outs' would call a faculty member to take care of their patients while they were in the hospital and the patients would go back to their regular pediatricians after they were discharged."[18]

The upside of this arrangement was that Christie was able to maintain control of the medicine being practiced on his ward. He could also ensure that his patients received top-quality care and that full-time faculty would not be distracted from their research interests. The downside of the situation, however, was that patient care sometimes lacked continuity. Perhaps more important, the arrangement served to feed Vanderbilt's reputation among the locals as an elitist institution manned by insensitive snobs.

Dr. James O'Neill, who was a young pediatric surgeon during Christie's reign, recalled there was another factor at work. Over the course of the years, Christie's budget for the entire pediatrics department hovered between only thirty-five thousand dollars and fifty thousand dollars. O'Neill said, "Vanderbilt doctors earned a pittance compared to community physicians, and Christie didn't particularly want that aired in the department. He kind of looked down on them, because he thought that he and his staff were purists."[19] The more outsiders he let in, the greater the chance that his own staff would abandon the academic mission for higher paying jobs.

Disease, however, doesn't wait for financial issues and crosstown arguments to be resolved. In the summer of 1948, Middle Tennessee was slammed with a severe epidemic of poliomyelitis. Christie petitioned for funds to create a special ward for all the polio cases that were pouring into Vanderbilt Hospital. Dean Goodpasture simply didn't have the resources or the nursing staff for such a unit. Desperately ill patients streamed in anyway, needing the kind of intensive care and elaborate equipment available only at a major medical center. Christie was going to have to ask private citizens for help.[20] Fortunately, the Junior League Home for Crippled Children was already in full swing, taking care of indigent polio patients who were well enough for convalescence. Vanderbilt was certain it could call on the Junior League. There was one minor hitch, however. Quite a few League members had personal and professional ties to physicians who'd been denied admitting privileges to Vanderbilt.

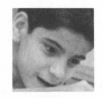

The Scourge of Polio | 6

"In those days physical therapy was thought of as a voodoo kind of thing. [Doctors] weren't threatened by it, they just thought it was a bunch of hogwash. They were only just beginning to understand that maybe this physical therapy was doing some good things for kids."

—Nelson Andrews, former member of the Junior Chamber of Commerce and early proponent of the Clinic Bowl

Polio was a hard thing to figure out," Sarah Sell noted. "It's a disease that enters through the gastrointestinal tract, but it produces its lesions in the spinal cord, and the sequelae [negative aftereffects] are neurological. It took us a long time to figure that out."

While she and other experts in infectious disease were trying to unravel the mystery of polio, the United States remained in the grips of an epidemic that would last from 1943 until 1956. Four hundred thousand people would be stricken and twenty-two thousand of them would die. Although only 1 percent of polio victims would be left paralyzed, the fact that there were no medicines to treat it and no real understanding of how it was spread made the disease all the more terrifying.[1] Teachers were afraid to accept the siblings of polio victims into their classrooms. Hospital dieticians were afraid to handle food trays that a polio patient might have touched. Janitors were afraid to clean their rooms. The disease knew no racial or socioeconomic lines; it affected people of all ethnicities and hit wealthy families as hard as poor ones.

Once scientists discovered that the poliomyelitis virus was spread by fecal-oral or oral-oral transmission, they could begin the search for a vaccine. That would take years.

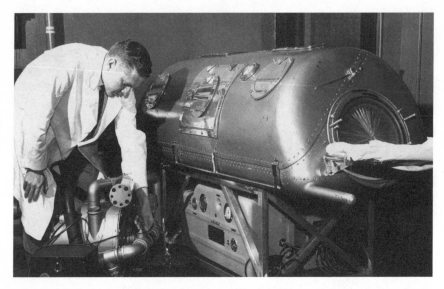

Dr. Randy Batson made improvements to the iron lung respirator that enabled many polio patients to breathe.

Vanderbilt became the primary care center for most of the polio cases in Tennessee and other areas of the South. Amos Christie secured a grant from the Tennessee chapter of the National Foundation for Infantile Paralysis (NFIP), later known as the March of Dimes, for Randy Batson to travel up to Boston for a postgraduate course in running respirators and caring for patients with severe paralytic polio. During the muggy summer months, they began a primitive form of triage in the emergency room. The pediatric resident would perform a spinal tap on the patients, many of whom had infections other than polio. (Some of those diseases were also life-threatening, but they were different problems altogether).[2] Only the paralyzed polio patients or those with respiratory complications were transferred up to the wards. The others were sent home with instructions for care.

Admission into the hospital marked the beginning of a complicated process. Respirators were scattered all over the facility, taking up space on both the pediatric and adult wards. During severe epidemics in Middle Tennessee, NFIP employees would scramble to bring in whatever respirators they could find anywhere in the country. Often the machines they would locate were broken or would malfunction as soon as they were plugged in, so a repairman had to stay on call at the hospital twenty-four hours a day during peak polio epidemics, which usually lasted from June through September. Without air-conditioning, the polio unit grew swelteringly hot and miserable.[3]

"Patients and staff were worn out from the heat," wrote Marjorie Mathias Dobbs, one of the Vanderbilt nurses on the polio unit. "Since the patients were completely dependent on the respirator, when we had a power failure, nurses, doctors, and other staff came from everywhere to hand pump each respirator."[4] During electrical outages, Christie would join his team in manually pumping the machines to keep patients alive.

At one point, Vanderbilt ran out of iron lung respirators and had to borrow an incubator and ventilation equipment from a local veterinarian in order to treat a sick baby.[5]

The iron lung respirator was draconian. Large and eerie, it enclosed the entire body. Only the patient's head and neck were exposed, surrounded by a collar that moved in and out with the respirator. Patients were in constant danger of having the skin on their necks rubbed raw from the friction created by the collar. With loud mechanical hisses and gasps, the machine essentially breathed for the patient. It exerted negative pressure to suck up the chest, thereby breathing in, and then cycled off to let the chest fall, thereby breathing out. Sixteen times a minute the process was repeated. Nurses and doctors had to stick their arms through tightly sealed portholes in order to deliver care.[6]

One of the first lessons learned by a Vanderbilt intern was how to transfer patients into an iron lung. In order for the students to understand just how confining and uncomfortable the respirator was for patients, Dr. J. C. Peterson made his interns climb inside one. He then turned the respirator on. "That machine breathed in and out whether you wanted it to or not," Sell recalled.[7]

The 1949 polio epidemic was an especially trying one and proved to be a rough initiation for Henry Clark as he began his new job as hospital director. In December of that year, however, he was able to announce to his overworked doctors and nurses, "In all, 104 patients, approximately 80 percent of all Middle Tennessee cases, were treated in this unit without a death. One polio patient died who had been transferred in critical condition from another hospital after the unit was closed."[8]

Given the state of disarray in treating polio patients, Christie determined that he had to create a special ward for their care. Yet he knew all too well that Vanderbilt was flat broke. So, he decided to appeal to a few community powerbrokers for help. Without asking permission from Goodpasture's successor, Dean John Youmans, Christie held a series of informal meetings with several of Nashville's more prominent philanthropists, including Mrs. Bernard "Leah Rose" Werthan, whose husband ran Werthan Bag Company; Sam Fleming, president of Third National Bank; and D. E. "Hap" Motlow, owner of the Jack Daniel Distillery. At the end of his meeting, Hap Motlow offered to take on the project alone, matching any funds Vanderbilt received from the NFIP. The Foundation would buy the necessary equipment, and Motlow would help pay construction costs.

Christie was delighted. Chancellor Branscomb, on the other hand, was livid. Once again, Christie had acted like a loose cannon, forgoing the chain of command in order to serve the immediate needs of his own department. With a wink, Christie later explained, "Timing and emotional appeal are large factors in fundraising." He also forgave Branscomb for the scolding.[9]

In 1953, Ward 3320 opened as a unit within pediatrics, dedicated strictly for polio patients, both children and adults, who would receive care free of charge. Randy Batson was named medical director and headed up the acquisition and refinement of respirators, while Pete Riley and Robert Merrill, who came a little later, ran the clinical service. Edith Fly, who had years of experience with polio patients, was named head nurse.[10] Only one of ten in the nation, the polio ward, which soon brought national acclaim to Vanderbilt Hospital, was officially titled the Regional Poliomyelitis Respiratory Center. Among Tennesseans, it earned the moniker Tank Town.

Tank Town was often one of the busiest wards in the hospital, with as many as twenty-five respirators of various types firing at once. Hundreds of patients would receive treatment there, with some forced to remain in an iron lung for two years or more. When patients first arrived, they were usually put into the iron lung for twenty-four hours a day, with the goal of weaning them off the respirators as soon as they developed the muscle capacity to breathe on their own. Gradually they were pulled off the iron lung for short periods of time each day and put on a more comfortable chest respirator. Eventually, they graduated to a rocking bed.[11]

Operating like a constantly moving seesaw, the rocking bed provided passive breathing by lowering the head of the bed and then raising it up to almost a standing position. The patients vastly

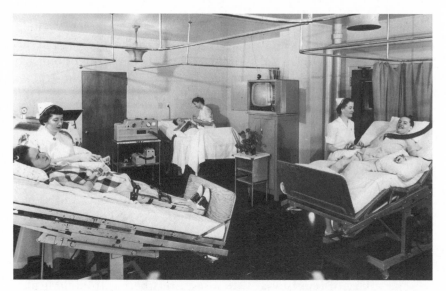

Vanderbilt's polio unit, with its rocking beds and various ventilation machines, became known locally as Tank Town.

preferred it to the iron lung machine, since they were simply strapped onto the bed without any accompanying appliances. The perpetual swaying took some adjustment. Still, wrote Marjorie Mathias Dobbs, "They felt free."[12]

Less than a year after opening, Tank Town had thirty-three patients successfully graduate from the ward. Most went home in time for Christmas.[13] The unit was also unique in the little luxuries it provided that couldn't be found on other floors of the hospital. Patients had access to air-conditioning, televisions, occupational therapy classes, and in the spring and summer, were taken outside for picnics. A nurse, a doctor, and an electrician accompanied each patient on these little outdoor treks.[14]

Henry Clark had already initiated the process of pulling Vanderbilt Hospital out of a financial quagmire. He was also a man of acute vision and innate instinct. He realized that Nashville was missing a specialty service that had already become popular in other parts of the country—physical therapy. Meharry Medical College's Hubbard Hospital was the only place in town offering its polio patients both medical treatment and physical therapy,[15] although the Junior League Home and a few other sanitaria had physical therapists on staff to work with patients. In other words, the people in town receiving sanctioned

physical therapy tended to be exclusively young, black, and/or indigent. Clearly, it was time for Vanderbilt to play catch up.

Vanderbilt had once had a physical therapy department but had
closed it during the war and never reopened it. "In those days
physical therapy was thought of as a voodoo kind of thing," explained
community leader Nelson Andrews. "[Doctors] weren't threatened by
it, they just thought it was a bunch of hogwash. They were only just
beginning to understand that maybe this physical therapy was doing
some good things for kids."[16]

Clark convinced Christie that the community was ready to unite
with Vanderbilt to control polio's devastation. He was right. They
worked out a deal with the Nashville Junior Chamber of Commerce
and Big Brothers to financially support a special physical therapy
unit. Vanderbilt, in turn, would provide space, maintenance, and
supervision. The National Foundation for Infantile Paralysis would
pay the salary of one physical therapist and the local public health
department would pay for another.[17] Christie had calculated they
could pay each therapist a salary based on the estimated number of
patient visits. Unfortunately, after all the tallying was done, the finan-
ciers figured they could afford about $3.05 per visit. So be it. They
sent an emissary up to Boston Children's Hospital in search of two

*In the spring and summer, doctors and nurses took Tank Town patients outdoors
for picnics.*

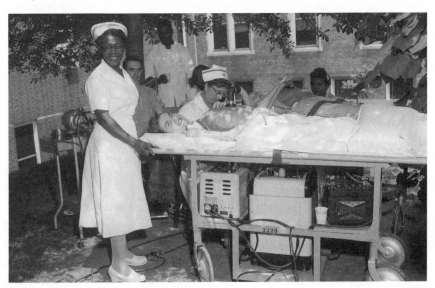

women, preferably young, unmarried, energetic, devoted to the cause, and willing to work for pennies.

At that time, the executive director of the Nashville chapter of the NFIP was Mrs. Percie Warner Lea, widow of Luke Lea, the former affluent publisher of the *Nashville Tennessean*. A decade earlier, her husband had been arrested and served time for business misdealings, only to be released two years later with a full pardon. Although Lea was able to repair his reputation, he would never regain his fortune or his health, and he died in 1945. In the late 1940s, at the age of fifty, his wife, Percie, needed to find a job. Having donated many volunteer hours and money to the National Foundation, she was soon hired by the local chapter to be its executive director, a position she took very seriously. Genteel, thin, and bird-like, Lea quietly and diplomatically commanded respect.[18] Among her many responsibilities, she took on the task of tracking down the perfect candidates to run Vanderbilt's physical therapy unit. She found them in Dorothy Fredrickson and Deborah Kinsman.

It's hard to understand why these two women would accept such a position, other than the allure of beginning something from scratch that would affect so many lives. In the summer of 1949, they drove down from Boston and entered Tennessee via old Route 70, "curving, climbing, or zooming downhill endlessly in the pouring rain."[19] Dr. Christie, Dr. Clark, Dr. Batson, and Dr. Robert Foote, representing the Crippled Children's division of the Tennessee Public Health Department, met them at their new office space—two rooms in the basement of what is now Vanderbilt's Medical Center North, where the old blood bank had once resided. The area was like a catacomb, dark and dingy, with exposed pipes running along the ceilings. Shortly afterwards, Lea took the two ladies shopping for equipment with no limit to their spending budget.[20] They arranged the basement rooms with ramps, bars, beds, mats, slings, and weights. In the early days, they'd work six days a week. After a year at Vanderbilt, they were allowed one Saturday off a month, and after several years, were finally given one full week's vacation.[21]

Despite these less-than-optimal conditions, Frederickson and Kinsman remained at Vanderbilt for the next thirty years. Some say they worked miracles. "I think many of us would not have survived had it not been for those two ladies," said Nickie Lancaster, who contracted polio during the 1949–50 epidemic. "They argued with the doctors and they chewed them out, and they fought to have them correct my body cast."[22]

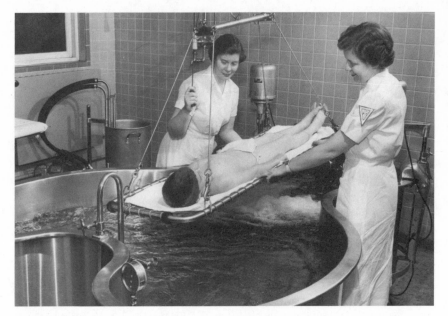

With financial backing from the National Foundation for Infantile Paralysis (later known as the March of Dimes), Vanderbilt opened a department of physical therapy, which improved the treatment options for patients with polio.

James O'Neill agreed that in their basement kingdom, Fredrickson and Kinsman reigned supreme. "Those two women had such great credibility that if they said a brace wasn't right, it got corrected," he said.[23]

O'Neill knew firsthand. In 1960, one week into the first year of his surgical residency at Vanderbilt, he contracted polio from one of his patients and was left paralyzed in his upper torso. He spent the next three years in rehabilitation. Orthopedic surgeon Dr. William Hillman fitted him with a custom-made brace that allowed him to use his arms and sent him down to physical therapy. With limited use of his arms and hands, O'Neill was certain that he would have to give up his dreams of becoming a surgeon. The physical therapists would have none of that. "You're going to get back to what you want to do!" they told him.

They made him work out harder and with more exertion than he thought possible, even calling his wife at night to be sure he was completing his home exercises. O'Neill said, "They knew how to be friendly and nice and gentle, and at other times how to be as tough as nails."[24]

O'Neill would indeed regain the function in all his affected muscles. In fact, the experience would guide him into a career as a pediatric surgeon. Later, he would become the director of surgical sciences at Vanderbilt.

Given that these two wonderful therapists had appeared in Nashville like a godsend, the Vanderbilt administration had to figure out how to continue supporting them. The year before their arrival, the Junior Chamber of Commerce had spearheaded a fund-raising campaign for the March of Dimes to benefit the building of Vanderbilt's physical therapy department. Members went door-to-door to neighborhood houses asking for change—hence, the "March of Dimes." The following year, more volunteers participated in the fund-raiser, embarking on a "one-night parents' march on polio, signaled by the blowing of whistles and sirens throughout the County."[25]

Another fund-raiser targeted many Tennesseans' favorite pastime. Tennesseans tend to measure the seasons of the year in relation to high school football. Up until that time, teams had never engaged in an end-of-season state high school football championship. Members of the Junior Chamber of Commerce came up with the idea to stage the Thanksgiving Day Clinic Bowl, a high school football tournament where the proceeds would support the Vanderbilt Physical Therapy department. The athletic event played right to Amos Christie's

The therapist closest to the respirator is Deborah Kinsman. Along with Dorothy Frederickson, she came to Vanderbilt in 1949 and worked as a physical therapist there for the next thirty years.

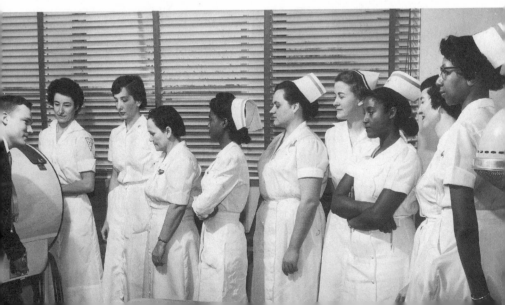

strengths. He was able to bolster his fame as a former Rose Bowl participant. Legendary sportswriter Fred Russell and his cronies gave the
games plenty of coverage in the local media. And Tennesseans were
able to extend their beloved sport that much longer into the season.

The Clinic Bowl was a huge success, raising ten thousand dollars
that first year (and ultimately raising more than five million dollars
over the course of its fifty-five-year history). Commented Christie,
"The Clinic Bowl . . . is the one thing which Vanderbilt does each year
which is not controversial."[26]

In the meantime, scientists around the globe were holed up in their
laboratories in a vigorous race to produce the first viable vaccine against
the poliomyelitis virus. One of these researchers was Jonas Salk. The son
of a New York City garment worker, Salk had become involved in the
development of a vaccine against influenza during World War II while
studying under famed virologist Thomas Francis Jr., at the University of
Michigan's School of Public Health. After the war ended, Salk moved to
the University of Pittsburgh School of Medicine and turned his attention
to polio. He received coveted funding from the NFIP and focused on
what was then considered a controversial technique for vaccine production: using a killed form of the virus to stimulate antibodies. Following a
few successful preclinical trials, Salk embarked on a daring test of his
research. With his respected mentor Dr. Thomas Francis in charge of
the design and evaluation of the double-blind field trials, 1.8 million
schoolchildren from the United States, Canada, and Finland were inocu-
lated with the Salk vaccine for poliomyelitis. On April 12, 1955, Francis
took to the airways, announcing to the public that the vaccine was "safe,
effective and potent."[27]

That same day at Vanderbilt, the physicians working on the polio
unit suspected some good news was coming. Christie, Batson, and
Riley jumped into Christie's car, and flew downtown, arriving at the
Noel Hotel in time to hear Dr. Francis's landmark pronouncement.
The United States had a polio vaccine. Finally.[28]

This was a spectacular moment for the three men. They returned
to the hospital, back to their patients wrapped in iron lungs, being
flipped up and down on rocking beds, struggling to walk in heavy
metal leg braces. The breakthrough was a preventative, however, and
not a cure, doing little to change the lives of those patients already
stricken. "VACCINE 'TRIUMPH' ENDS POLIO THREAT," trum-
peted headlines of papers across North America.[29] They would not
be accurate. The threat, albeit lessened, still continued. April 12, 1955,

was only day one. It would be many more years before Tank Town would close.

After the release of the Salk vaccine, cases of poliomyelitis began to drop precipitously. But scientists soon ran into a roadblock—the vaccine's effectiveness didn't last. As a result, some people who'd had one shot and thought they were immune still contracted the virus. Vanderbilt's surgery resident James O'Neill was one such case. Public health officials had to refine their vaccination plan to include a three-shot regimen of the killed virus. Such a regimen compounded problems of access, particularly for states with large rural populations like Tennessee.

In the first three years after the Salk vaccine hit the market, the incidence of polio in Tennessee was 19.1 per 100,000 citizens. The rate in 1958 was 3.3 per 100,000 people. On closer examination, however, officials discovered that some counties had a vaccination rate of 75 percent, while others struggled by with a 17 percent vaccination rate.[30] In other words, the burden of disease was largely borne in the remote, impoverished counties. Plus, many of those infected had the paralytic form of the disease, so the patients being transferred to Tank Town were extremely sick.

Even more disturbing, an epidemic broke out in the summer of 1959, primarily among children who had received partial immunization. In August, the state recorded eighty cases, compared to thirty-five cases a year earlier.[31] People feared polio was on the upsurge again.

Relief finally came in the shape of a sugar cube. Dr. Albert Sabin of the Cincinnati College of Medicine had been none too pleased that he had lost the vaccine marathon to Jonas Salk, and he continued to believe that immunization could be delivered in a more convenient form. In 1957, he offered Randy Batson some of the oral vaccine he was working on to see if children responded in preclinical trials. As opposed to Salk's killed virus vaccine, Sabin's technique used a live attenuated vaccine that could be taken by mouth rather than through a shot. Christie, Batson, and Dr. William Cheatham were part of a team that helped show that the oral polio vaccine worked in children and was much easier to give to large numbers of people.[32]

"We covered such a wide area that we always had more patients than we could deal with. In 1959 we had a lot of patients," said Robert Merrill. "Then the Sabin vaccine came into use. The number of our cases went from sixty to four. So I saw the impact of the Sabin vaccine. I don't care who's applying for sainthood, it was the Sabin vaccine that made the difference."[33]

By the mid-1950s, the menace of polio, while still present, began to wane. At the Junior League Home for Crippled Children, the patient census of polio-stricken children began to decline. Concurrently, a novel concept was infiltrating the American approach to convalescence. Medical personnel started to question the dogma of separating young children from their parents while they recovered from a major illness. Perhaps, they suggested, even poor children should be allowed to stay with their families as much as possible. Responding to this notion, providers began to make health care more transportable and more adaptable to a home environment. Also, in the

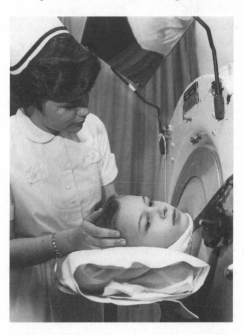

wake of such crises as World War II and various polio epidemics, improvements in orthopedic medicine were booming, thanks to contributions by dedicated physicians and engineers. As a result, those children admitted into the Junior League Home had shorter stays. In the first half of the century, the average stay for a child had been eighteen months. By 1958, it had dropped to thirty days.

The sum total of these three phenomena—a polio vaccine, an emphasis on home convalescence, and advances in orthopedic medicine—forced the members of the Junior League of Nashville to reassess their relationship

Although the Salk polio vaccine was a medical breakthrough, Vanderbilt was still treating a large number of polio patients into the late 1950s, until the Sabin vaccine helped eradicate the disease in America.

with the facility that they'd founded, loved, and nurtured for thirty-five years. Had the time come, they wondered, to finally close the Junior League Home for Crippled Children? As it so happened, the local women of the National Council of Jewish Women helped them reach a decision.

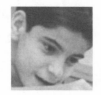

Nashville's Jewish Community Weighs In | 7

"This represents the highest type of public service and the children of Nashville as well as the members of the staffs of the various hospitals and the Pediatric Society are eternally indebted to you and to the members of your organization . . . I cannot help but think of the Council Home, as far as I am personally concerned, as the Vanderbilt Pediatric Department Convalescent Home."

—Dr. Amos Christie, regarding the Convalescent Home for Children, in a correspondence to the Nashville Section of the National Council of Jewish Women

In the late 1950s, two of Nashville's most active civic organizations, the Junior League and the Council of Jewish Women, arrived almost simultaneously at a crossroads that forced them to reexamine their key projects. With its patient census dropping at the Home for Crippled Children since the introduction of the polio vaccine, the Junior League of Nashville initiated a series of meticulous studies during 1957 and 1958 to determine the health and welfare needs of orthopedically challenged children in Middle Tennessee and how the stated mission of the Home could be adapted to help.

League members first voted to raise the income level of qualifying families so that indigent patients still had priority, but nonindigent children could also be admitted. The League also studied the practicality of building a separate children's hospital in town, but immediately dropped the idea, believing that project was far beyond the group's scope or capability.

Several other items from the studies remained on the table, however, ripe for further investigation. These included raising the maximum age of admission from fourteen to sixteen; broadening the diagnostic categories to cover severely emotionally disturbed children, victims of abuse, and children with cardiovascular illnesses or acute trauma; admitting black children as inpatients; expanding the Home's geographic territory; and combining forces with another local facility, the Convalescent Home for Children run by the Nashville Section of the National Council of Jewish Women.[1] The resolution to this last issue would become a cornerstone in the founding of the Vanderbilt Children's Hospital.

The League and the Council had run parallel operations since 1947. The idea for the Council's Home was sparked in 1943, after Nashville Mayor Thomas Cummings had convened representatives from the city's most prominent civic, medical, and religious organizations to hear a desperate plea for assistance from the Davidson County Public Health Department. At that time, Director Dr. John Lentz told the group that while Middle Tennessee offered many health care services, there was no place where impoverished children could recuperate from major medical illnesses. The Junior League

These 1948 board members of the Nashville Section of the National Council of Jewish Women were responsible for the opening and operation of the group's Convalescent Home for Children.

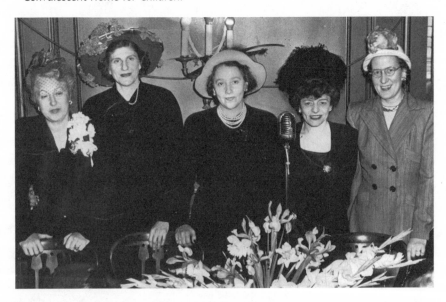

Home was designed to accommodate orthopedic rehabilitation only. Local hospitals were overburdened with children suffering from noninfectious diseases who were well enough to be discharged but too sick to return to less-than-optimal home environments, Lentz explained. These children were on the mend from rheumatic fever, chorea[2], nephritis, malnutrition, and emotional impairments—all of which required a safe, healthy atmosphere for recovery.[3]

The president of the local Council of Jewish Women, Elizabeth Lowenheim Jonas (later Jacobs), attended that meeting, bringing with her another Council member, Leah Belle Eskind. Eskind's son had once been deathly ill and she vowed that if he survived, she was going to "give one thousand dollars to start something for children." After hearing Lentz's speech, she realized she had found her cause. "I'll give one thousand dollars to start it," she announced, thereby committing the Council to the project.[4]

Elizabeth Jacobs responded as all good presidents do—she immediately began to delegate. Somebody had to conduct a survey of local facilities, doctors, nurses, hospitals, and charitable organizations to determine exactly what the needs were and what the costs might be. She assigned that task to Leah Rose Werthan.

Werthan and her husband, Bernard, were already well-established philanthropists in Nashville by that time, as was the extended Werthan family. She had graduated from Wellesley College intending to become a doctor, but had given up those dreams when she married. During World War II, like Hortense Ingram and other civic-minded women, she had volunteered as a nurse's aide at Vanderbilt Hospital. After the war ended, fascinated by medical science, she continued to volunteer as a receptionist in Vanderbilt's Tumor Clinic. There she met a little boy from an outlying county who had a large melanoma on his hand. His doctors debated for several days and finally decided to amputate the boy's hand—to be followed by daily courses of outpatient radiation. The child's family would have to travel back and forth about one hundred miles a day for the treatment. By then Werthan had grown attached to the boy and to his family and was convinced that what they and other families were going through—in fact, the whole state of convalescent care in Nashville—was totally unacceptable. She would personally have to fix that.[5]

The Council, under Werthan's chairmanship, spent the next four years conducting research and developing plans for a convalescent facility for children with noncontagious diseases, receiving endorsements by the Nashville Academy of Medicine, the Davidson County Medical Society, and all the local social service agencies that dealt with children. These women found that each year as many as three hundred of the city's indigent children were repeatedly hospitalized for the same illness because they couldn't access convalescent care after being discharged.[6]

While surveying local physicians, Werthan made an appointment to speak with Dr. Barney Brooks, the curmudgeonly head of the Department of Surgery at Vanderbilt, a doctor she'd seen in action during her stint as a volunteer. He was, she said, "a very brilliant, competent, nasty man." Werthan believed that Brooks's opinion and insight about surgical issues would be crucial as plans moved forward. When she explained her agenda about the Home, he said that he thought it was a splendid idea.

"But," he told her, "I want to give you one piece of advice. Don't put the name 'Jewish' in at all. Just leave it out."

"Why do you say that, Dr. Brooks?" she asked.

"Because you'll do better," he answered.

Bristling with indignation, Werthan told him:

> We have every intention of naming it the Council of Jewish Women's Home for Convalescent Children. And, Dr. Brooks, let me tell you something. Don't you ever make any remark like that until you're a Jew. And if you're a Jew, or if you become a Jew, then you'll understand what you're saying. But until you do, don't you ever say anything like that to me or to any other Jew. It's very unbecoming![7]

She then turned and walked out of his office.

Leah Rose Werthan, like her husband, belonged to a Jewish family that had lived in Nashville since the middle of the 1800s. During that period, Nashville had nurtured a small but adamantine population of born-and-bred, well-established Southern Jews. Most of these were families of German extraction, who immigrated to the United States and moved into the South to take advantage of business opportunities in the smaller cities. They stayed there, forming modest-sized Jewish communities and often quickly assimilated into the local society.

The first identifiable community of Jewish citizens in Nashville began around 1851, consisting of "five families and eight young men."[8] During the Civil War, like many Tennesseans, sons and brothers joined armies on both sides of the conflict. At least twenty Jewish men from Nashville fought for the Confederacy.[9] If they were dubious about which side to join, however, Ulysses S. Grant, serving as the commander of the Department of Tennessee, helped them make up their minds. In 1862, when Grant's Union forces occupied the city, he became frustrated by the number of merchants applying for trade permits, which he believed were responsible for the rampant black market in cotton. If they were merchants, he reasoned, they must be Jews. In November of that year he issued the following:

> Give orders to all the conductors on the road that no Jews are to be permitted to travel on the railroad southward from any point. They may go north and be encouraged in it; but they are such an intolerable nuisance that the department must be purged of them.[10]

By the following month, Grant's outrage was unbounded, and he issued to his underlings what historians would refer to as "the infamous General Order No. 11," demanding that all Jews from Kentucky, Mississippi, and Tennessee be expelled from the area within twenty-four hours after receipt of the order.

Jewish soldiers and supporters of the Union were incensed by the decree. Fortunately for them, however, by 1862 quite a few Jewish men had lived in the area for at least a decade and were respected as merchants, professionals, and humanitarians in their local communities. News about the expulsion flamed across the country.

In his office in Washington, D.C., President Lincoln was inundated with a backlash of telegrams and letters. Jewish leaders in St. Louis, Louisville, and Cincinnati staged organized protests.

Shortly, Lincoln sent a message to Grant, strongly suggesting that the general revoke No. 11—which he did three days later.[11]

Because they'd had to fight for the right to live and work in their home states, these Jewish sons-of-the-South became that much more devoted to and entrenched in the social fabric of their cities. They were permanent citizens, interested in local issues like education, the arts, and public health; they were aware that through acts of generosity they became more valued and appreciated within their hometowns. They were also slogging through Reconstruction side by side with their fellow Nashvillians. According to Jewish historian, Feodora S. Frank, "During the years 1870–1901, Jew and Gentile worked together, attended school together, supported public and civic movements, but walked their religious and social paths separately. There was very little of anti-Semitism evident in Nashville during these years."[12]

By the turn of the twentieth century, Nashville's Jewish population faced a new challenge—assimilating an influx of Eastern European refugees into their tight-knit society. Whereas the existing families tended to be well-educated and middle- or upper-class, the new arrivals from Russia spoke no English, had little money, and often were without formal education.[13] Nashville's Jews, who by then were steeped in Southern gentility, were taken aback by the crude, rough-edged manners and attitudes of their Eastern European brethren.

The women of the city felt obligated to help the immigrants adapt to their new country. In 1901, they formed a Nashville Section of the National Council of Jewish Women, chartered as "a volunteer organization, inspired by Jewish values, that works through a program of research, education, advocacy, and community service, to improve the quality of life for women, children and families and strives to ensure individual rights and freedom for all."[14] To that end, its sixty founding members established a kindergarten, a social house, and a

Leah Rose Werthan, an active philanthropist in the Nashville community, was instrumental in founding the National Council of Jewish Women's Convalescent Home for Children, which opened in 1947. Photo by Don Cravens, Nashville Tennessean, *November 23, 1947.*

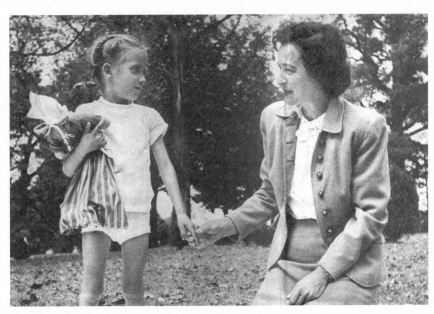

settlement center for the incoming citizens. Through the efforts of the Council, the immigrants learned trades, went to school, and were taught to speak English.[15]

As the decades progressed, the Council took on more and more community projects, and by the end of World War II, had become the Jewish women's counterpart to the Junior League of Nashville. Both groups were comprised largely of college-educated women who were unafraid of social activism for the betterment of their communities. Which is why Dr. John Lentz had such a receptive audience when he made his appeal for a convalescent home.

The Council membership numbered over six hundred women by the 1940s, and they were capable of exerting immeasurable influence and peer pressure. Knowing they had to have start-up funds to get the Home off the ground, they sponsored a one-night-only fund-raising dinner at the Woodmont Country Club. In that single evening in 1945, the Jewish citizens of Nashville pledged seventy-four thousand dollars in seed money. Within two years the Council had raised one hundred twenty thousand dollars, including an initial grant from the Nashville Community Chest, the first time that charity had provided financial support to a recipient before it had even been in operation.[16, 17]

With a hefty start-up bank account, Leah Rose Werthan knew what kind of building they could afford. She was on the verge of signing a contract for a donated tract of property in West Nashville when she received a phone call telling her about an ad for a house being put on the market in a fire sale. Located on Vultee Boulevard off of Murfreesboro Pike, it included a building and twenty-two acres of land. The only catch was that the contract had to be drawn up and signed immediately.

Werthan drove over to investigate. When she got there, she was met by a charming man by the name of Dr. Abt, an alleged theosophist, or proponent of the philosophy that through knowledge of God one can achieve spiritual ecstasy. Abt, it turned out, was actually operating a peculiar kind of sanitarium for alcoholics. Werthan walked in and faced a parade of filthy men lying around in cots, wrapped in stinking, brown khaki blankets that were soaked in alcohol. They were receiving Abt's special "cure."

She explained, "He put them on this cot and they lived under those smelly blankets and drank all they could get in their system, until they got really sick and then eventually they were supposed to be cured."[18]

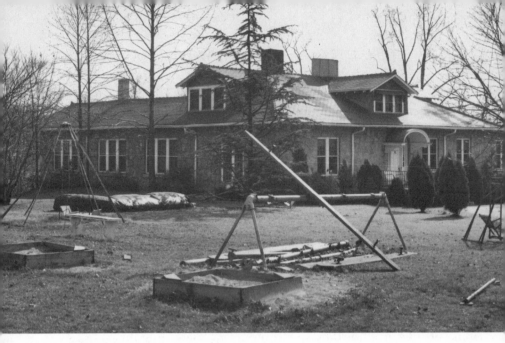

Nashville's National Council of Jewish Women purchased twenty-two acres and a house on Vultee Boulevard and converted it into a convalescent home for children with noncontagious medical problems. Photo by Ralph Starr, Nashville Banner, *March 1949.*

Abt was in a hurry. The Tennessee legislature had recently passed an ordinance outlawing any quack doctors who'd been posing as theosophists, forcing them to leave the state. He told her that he needed a contract by the next morning and he wanted a check for the downpayment that afternoon—a Saturday. Excitedly, she called the Woodmont Country Club and sent a messenger to pull the men on the Home Board advisory committee off the golf course. By the following day, Abt had split town with a check for forty-two thousand dollars, leaving behind a large chunk of property, a nice-sized house, and a basement stacked floor-to-ceiling with boxes, crates, and cartons of whiskey.[19]

While contractors were renovating the facility into a twenty-bed convalescent home, two hundred women of the Council attended volunteer training classes so they could serve as dieticians, gray lady service volunteers, nurses, as well as transportation, administrative, and clerical aides. The Council hired registered nurse Miss Isabel Jones in the dual position of superintendent and head nurse, in addition to two practical nurses and a social worker. The state of Tennessee provided a teacher, who came three days a week, and Amos Christie supplied a senior medical student from Vanderbilt who lived on-site and was on twenty-four-hour call. Dr. Harry Estes donated his services as the Home's consulting physician and other local doctors rotated through to see patients.[20] In any given month, the referring physicians might include Robert Merrill and Pete Riley of Vanderbilt, Thomas Frist Sr., Thomas Zerfoss Jr., Lindsay Bishop, Luther Beazley of Donelson, and Julian Gant of Madison.[21]

Every child who was ambulatory was given an annual dental checkup. Each year, Al Menah Shriners with clowns and acrobats from the Shrine Circus made a special visit to the children in the Home. Minnie Pearl became a favorite guest entertainer and presented each child with a little radio.[22] Because the Council Home was nonsectarian, local ministers and priests volunteered to hold Sunday morning worship services, and various church groups sponsored Christmas and Easter parties for the patients. In deference to the Home's nonsectarian standing, Reverend James Reed Cox, pastor of the Tulip Street Methodist Church, explained that he designed his services "to lift up underlying principles of character and good citizenship, faith in God and in worship of one Father of us all."[23]

Unlike the Junior League Home, the National Council of Jewish Women's Home became intricately linked with the Vanderbilt pediatric department. Amos Christie sang its praises time and again on behalf of the university and of the Nashville Pediatric Society, of which

Every year, the Al Menah Shriners sent Shrine Circus performers to entertain the children at the Council of Jewish Women's Convalescent Home. Photo by Vernon Fox, Nashville Banner, *June 24, 1949.*

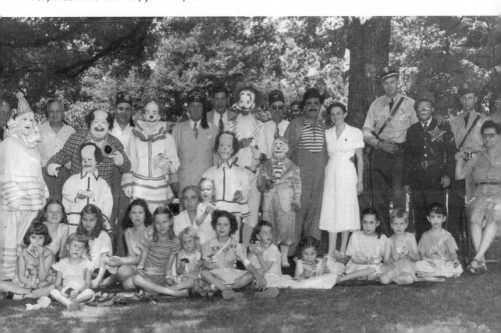

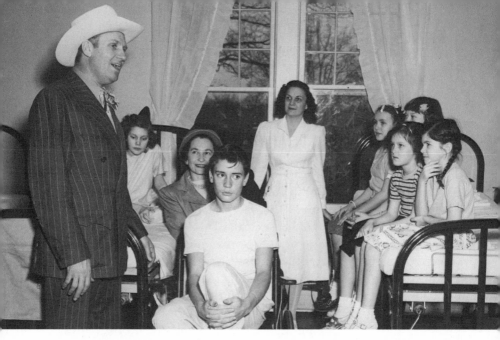

*Musical celebrities, such as Gene Autry (pictured) and Minnie Pearl, often enter-
tained the young patients at the Convalescent Home. President and founder Leah
Rose Werthan (wearing a hat) is behind the boy in the wheelchair. Photo by Ralph
Starr,* Nashville Banner, *February 25, 1949.*

he was president. " . . . This represents the highest type of public
service and the children of Nashville as well as the members of the
staffs of the various hospitals and the Pediatric Society are eternally
indebted to you and to the members of your organization," he wrote
to the Council officers, adding later, "I cannot help but think of the
Council Home, as far as I am personally concerned, as the Vanderbilt
Pediatric Department Convalescent Home."[24]

After a peak census in 1951, the number of patients admitted to
the Home began to steadily decline in the mid-1950s. Christie
explained to the women of the Council that antibiotics and modern
therapy had led to a general decrease in the demand for hospital
admissions and an upswing in outpatient treatment. In addition,
doctors were beginning to focus on preventive practices, such as
vaccines, which were resulting in fewer cases of acute disease. This
meant they were turning their attention to chronic illnesses.

Despite these ongoing transformations, Christie was not willing to
break his treasured bond with the Council Home. He told them:

> I do believe that in the future we will be asking you to allow our
> students and our house officers for additional opportunities to
> observe chronic illness at the convalescent homes and in this way

increase their usefulness for teaching purposes. You will then be completing the cycle of service for which we all strive, that is, community service, teaching and research.[25]

Alongside the dramatic changes happening in the medical world, equally profound events were occurring in society at large—although many people failed to see the connection. On May 17, 1954, the U.S. Supreme Court voted unanimously in its landmark ruling, *Brown v. Board of Education*, that laws maintaining separate schools for black and white students were inherently unconstitutional. Later the Supreme Court added that local, segregated school districts should proceed "with all deliberate speed" to implement their individual plans for desegregation.

After several years of heated negotiation, Nashville's political leaders devised a slow-drip solution—desegregation would begin with children entering first grade in 1957 and continue along year-by-year, achieving full integration by 1968. They labeled it the Nashville Plan. It never worked as intended.[26]

One consequence of *Brown v. Board of Education*, on the other hand, was that it jolted the sensibilities of many Southerners who had never really thought about the racial divisions in their communities. Beginning in 1956, the Executive Committee of Nashville's Council of Jewish Women began to suggest that they should strike the word "white" from the bylaws of the Home—as in, the Home is open to "white children, ages 2 to 16 . . ." Council members were not opposed to opening the Home to black children, they just weren't sure how to go about it gracefully. Should they make an announcement? Should they inform the parents of white children admitted to the Home? Should they actively recruit black patients? Flummoxed, they tabled the motion.[27]

However, every month the issue flared up again. Finally, the Council decided to wait on the ruling from the State Board of Education, which they hoped would provide guidance. Unfortunately, the delay gave hatemongers time to act. Late one September night, somebody dynamited the Hattie Cotton Elementary School, where one black child had previously enrolled. Nobody was hurt, but an entire wing of the building was destroyed.

Shortly afterwards, the national headquarters of the Jewish Women's Council got involved by asking its Southern chapters how they were handling integration issues. The Nashville Section

members responded with a lengthy explanation about the dilemma.
They described the state's actions to date and then added:

> . . . With regard to Nashville—Progress has been made in
> promoting racial good will. Many organizations have already
> become interracial, such as the League of Women Voters, the
> A.A.U.W., the United Churchwomen, the Nashville Academy of
> Medicine and the Davidson County Medical Society, and several
> others. Our Council of Community Agencies has for some years been
> interracial, we have Negro City Council members, Negro city school
> board members, Negro policemen and mailmen.[28]

By that time, the Council had spent two years working on race
relation issues with local leaders and had promoted, as a group, the
concept of integration. However, at a previous workshop attended by
both whites and blacks, participants returned to the parking lot and
discovered anti-desegregation pamphlets deposited on their cars and
the air let out of their cars' tires. Several members later received
threatening phone calls.

The Nashville Council concluded its response to the national
organization by stating, in essence, that they were cognizant of the
urgency of the issues and doing their best to find workable solutions.[29]

By 1957, many members of the Nashville Council believed that
their involvement in the Convalescent Home had run its course.
Patient numbers were down, many of the patients who did come to
the Home were so sick that they would not survive, and many of the
Jewish families in town had moved to the suburbs. Transporting
patients across town from Murfreesboro Pike to area hospitals and
back for clinic appointments had become incredibly inconvenient.
Few volunteers were willing to do that much driving. Representatives
from both the Council and the Junior League, which had always
maintained friendly relations, met to discuss common problems, but
had not come up with solid answers.

Council members decided that after a successful ten-year run, it
was time to turn operation of the Home over to a suitable community
organization. A committee from the Council met with the Junior
League's study group to discuss the possibility of combining the two
convalescent homes.

Then in March of 1958, racial tensions slammed home. A round of
dynamite exploded at the Jewish Community Center on West End

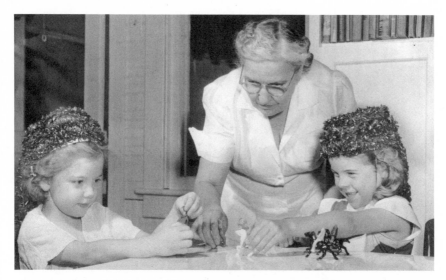

In 1958, after the Junior League of Nashville broadened its definition of the "crippled child," the remaining patients at the Council of Jewish Women's Home were transferred over to the Junior League Home and former head nurse Isabel Jones was given an extra month's pay for her devotion to duty. Photo by Bill Preston, Nashville Tennessean.

Avenue, followed by a phone threat to Rabbi William Silverman. He was warned that other Jewish interests would be targeted, along with "every other nigger-loving place or nigger-loving person in Nashville." Rabbi Silverman had been a vocal proponent of integration and had allowed interracial groups to hold meetings at the Jewish Community Center.[30] The threat shocked a city that had always appeared blanketed in harmony. The Council of Jewish Women, shaken but undeterred, pushed on to find a new overseer for their young patients.

In May of 1958, the Council received a reply from the Junior League stating that, after careful study, they would not be able to take in the Council Home's children because of a new admission policy and a reduction in the number of available beds.[31] Despite the setback, Council members decided to move ahead with plans to transfer the Home into new hands. A few months later, the Junior League had a change of heart and contacted the executives of the Council. The League had chosen to broaden the definition of the "crippled child," and would now accept children with medical as well as orthopedic needs. The Council put forth a recommendation to close the Council Home for Convalescent Children and allow the Junior League Home

for Crippled Children to accept those patients who met their newly
expanded admission requirements. By early November 1958, the
transfer was completed. The Junior League women took whatever
items in the Home's inventory they could use and the rest were
donated to various charitable agencies. In gratitude for their "devotion
to duty," nurse Isabel Jones and other workers were given an extra
month's pay.[32]

Finally, before the merger took place, Nashville's Council of
Jewish Women voted to remove the word "white" from the decade-
old bylaws that had governed their Home for Convalescent
Children.[33] It was a symbolic gesture, to be sure—but a significant
one, all the same.

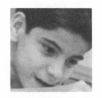

The Right Thing To Do | 8

"I think Nashville has always worked gradually towards change."

—Frances Jackson, former president of the Junior League of Nashville

The merger of the Council of Jewish Women's Convalescent Home with the Junior League of Nashville's Home for Crippled Children meant that Amos Christie and the pediatric house staff at Vanderbilt Medical School suddenly had a much cozier connection to the Junior League than ever before. Heretofore, Christie and the League ladies had been gracious and courteous to one another, but the orthopedists and private pediatricians in town had handled the bulk of medical needs of their patients. With the League's decision to expand the definition of the crippled child to include children with medical problems, the Vanderbilt Pediatrics Department, by default, would have to become more involved.

Dr. Ethel Walker, a Nashville-born pediatrician who had trained with Christie at Johns Hopkins, and, in fact, had served as the first female chief resident of pediatrics there, had taken on the responsibility of physician-in-charge at the Crippled Children's Home. She, like the other physicians who saw patients there, offered her services pro bono. Walker was a graduate of Vanderbilt Medical School, a longtime resident of Belle Meade, and a member of the Junior League. They were her people. Unlike the struggling, underpaid university physicians, she was in her comfort zone with League ladies. Three evenings a week, she rounded at the Home, often with a Vanderbilt resident or two in tow.

Although Christie had granted Walker admitting privileges at Vanderbilt, they maintained a somewhat frosty relationship. One day a week, the pediatric department held grand rounds from 8:00 until 9:00 in the morning. Ethel Walker, on the other hand, had a policy that she would sit at her telephone each morning from 7:30 until 8:30 a.m. so that parents could call to ask questions about their children. That way she could streamline her night call by encouraging parents to simply wait to speak with her until the next morning. Unfortunately, this policy meant that she was always late to grand rounds. Walker repeatedly asked Christie to hold grand rounds later in the morning, and Christie repeatedly insisted that she change her at-home call schedule. Neither doctor budged.[1]

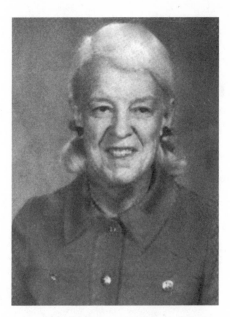

Dr. Ethel Walker, a resident of Belle Meade and a member of the Junior League, was the primary attending physician at the Home for Crippled Children.

Ethel Walker was the only child of a prominent Nashville attorney. She was also an avid fan of Vanderbilt basketball, and she often took her mother with her to the games. However, she ran such a rigid practice that parents were afraid to make a move without her consent. One night while she was at a basketball game, a worried mother called the house and Walker's father answered the phone.

"Oh, I just must ask her something! I just must ask her something!" said the frantic mom.

"I'm sorry she's not here," answered Mr. Walker.

"Well," the woman said, "maybe you can tell me . . . does castor oil mix with aspirin?"

The old gentleman pondered for a minute. "I'm not in any way a medical person," he replied, "so I'm not capable in any sort of way to give you a medical answer. But I can tell you one thing—as far as the state of Tennessee is concerned, there's no law against it!"[2]

Later, when friction developed between Christie and the Junior League, Walker was one of the Vanderbilt-appointed pediatricians who boldly sided with the League and against the Chief.

From the late 1950s until 1970, the leadership at the Junior League of Nashville hit its apex in terms of local influence. The organization had won the adoration of Middle Tennesseans for its good works, and the women who took charge of it year after year during that decade were resolute, dynamic, and surprisingly forward thinking, in that they were willing to push the established boundaries in a small Southern city that held steadfast to tradition. Many of these women had graduated from Vanderbilt and as undergraduates had joined the elite sororities of Kappa Alpha Theta (Theta) or Delta Delta Delta (Tri-Delt).

After World War II, Vanderbilt University had assumed the mantle of a party school and was renowned for its Greek life and panty raids.[3] Yet, in truth, sorority involvement provided many young women with invaluable skills for an evolving society. Although not their primary focus, sororities had begun participating in civic events that served the less fortunate. Members were forced to work together towards common goals. That meant negotiating, networking,

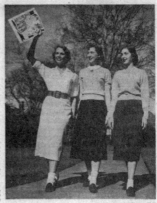

Pretty VU Coed Newshawks To Sell Tabloids Sunday

Three of Nashville's prettiest newshawks put their heads together yesterday and discussed newspapers, the weather and clothes—in that order.

The newshawks — girls from Vanderbilt university sororities—will be among the hundreds of Middle Tennessee volunteers who will sell THE NASHVILLE TENNESSEAN Crippled Children's tabloid Sunday morning. Proceeds from the tabloid sale will be used to support the Junior League Home for Crippled Children, at 2400 White ave., during the coming year.

The three Vanderbilt coeds are ll veterans of previous sales campaigns. In fact it will be the 16th one pretty Elise Dobson has sold he tabloids and she's only a freshman.

"Well, I was only 2 the first time sold them," she grinned. "My mother really did most of the work. But every year since then ve been out bright and early."

Elise, 18, daughter of Mr. and Mrs. Howard M. Dobson of Woodmont boulevard, discussed the rapidly approaching tabloid sale with Evelyn Gowdy, 20, a junior from Anchorage, Ky., and Salter Neal, 22, a senior from Carthage. It will be Evelyn's little sale and alter's fourth in Nashville. She lded the drive in Carthage before oming to Vanderbilt.

Weather Discussed

The weather entered the picture the girls discussed their plans or Sunday. What would it be ike? Therefore, what to wear?

"I've sold tabloids in every sort of weather," Elise reflected. "Hot, cold, rain, sleet—you name it. But I always enjoyed it. I seldom worry about what to wear—I'm always too steady that early in the morning.

(Continued on Page 9, Column 1)

—Staff photo by Jimmy Holt
Three of Vanderbilt university's prettiest sorority girls practice hawking THE NASHVILLE TENNESSEAN Shrine-Junior League tabloid. Elise Dobson, Pi Beta Phi, of Woodmont boulevard, waves an advance copy in the traditional style. With her, from left, are Salter Neal, Delta Delta Delta from Carthage, Tenn., and Evelyn Gowdy, Kappa Alpha Theta from Anchorage, Ky.

The caption to this 1957 photo reads: "Three of Vanderbilt university's prettiest sorority girls practice hawking the Nashville Tennessean Shrine–Junior League tabloid. . . ." *They are (left to right): Elise Dobson, Pi Beta Phi; Salter Neal, Delta Delta Delta; and Evelyn Gowdy, Kappa Alpha Theta. Photo by Jimmy Holt,* Nashville Tennessean, *April 10, 1957.*

researching facts before making decisions, and battling ideas through to consensus. Also, these young women figured out the structures and channels they'd need to traverse in order to succeed in their mission.

When they left college and joined the Junior League, they used these same skills, now finely honed, to make an impact on their community.

"I don't think it entered any of our minds that we couldn't do anything we set out to do," said Vanderbilt alumna and former Junior League President Mary Stumb.[4]

In 1960, sheltered from the outside world, Vanderbilt students were largely unaware that the metropolis surrounding their campus had become a virtual tinderbox.[5] African Americans were getting tired of the barriers and disparities they faced every time they tried to get ahead. The Nashville Plan for desegregating the public schools was creeping along ineffectively, and the educational gap between blacks and whites loomed large and ugly. Vanderbilt had limited its admission of black students to the Graduate, Law, and Divinity Schools, and even then had restricted them from dining in the cafeteria or playing intramural sports alongside white students. Downtown merchants allowed, even encouraged, black citizens to shop in their stores, but prohibited them from eating at their lunch counters.

Although black community leaders such as Robert Lillard, Avon Williams Jr., and Z. Alexander Looby had begun bridging the divide between minority concerns and the white establishment, they couldn't stem the tensions gurgling beneath the calm. An explosion was bound to happen.

By the century's sixth decade, Fisk University, Tennessee State University, American Baptist Theological Seminary, and Meharry Medical School had already educated a critical mass of black individuals who'd become part of the professional workforce. Members of the black middle class were tired of Tennessee's social inequities, both stated and implied. White and black community leaders were attending interracial meetings, but the pace was too slow for the existing group of idealistic black students at local universities. They were smart enough not to expect unanimity from the white community, but they knew they needed just enough support to tip the scales.

For several years, an underground civil rights movement had been brewing among the young and educated on various college campuses around Nashville. Among the planners was an African American student at Vanderbilt's Divinity School named James Lawson. Trained in the techniques of nonviolent protests, he began holding workshops in the basement of one of the local churches. He taught his followers how to engage in peaceful civil disobedience, how to dodge blows, and how to resist the impulse to respond to violence with violence. He and other leaders of the movement, such as John Lewis and Diane Nash, began to carefully plot their strategy of quiet rebellion.

However, on February 1, 1960, four freshman students at North Carolina A & T College touched off a rash of sit-ins across the South by seating themselves, on a whim, at the lunch counters at a Woolworth's store in Greensboro, North Carolina. The Nashville students were immediately energized to stage their own protests, eager to tap into the rapt attention the media was paying to racial discrimination. On February 13, 124 college students, the majority of whom were black, gathered downtown and seated themselves at the counters of local merchandisers. The storeowners closed the counters. Five days later, over 200 students infiltrated other lunch counters, costing the merchants precious business. Day after day, wave after wave, more students joined in; they moved through the downtown lunch counters, filled the jails, disrupted commerce, and agitated the city leaders who'd been trying to creep forward towards racial serenity. White hecklers began showing up at the sit-ins, screaming epithets and beating the students. The police arrived and arrested the orderly protesters for disorderly conduct. All the while, TV cameras captured images for the nation to see of well-dressed, soft-spoken African Americans being pummeled and harassed in Nashville by hate-filled, trash-mouthed whites as policemen and reporters looked on.

In early March, James Lawson and other black leaders met with Mayor Ben West to discuss an acceptable resolution to the protests. Lawson, who had counseled students but never personally partici-pated in the sit-ins, stepped forward to claim that the ordinance shop owners were using to close their lunch counters was a gimmick to suppress the protesters' right to be there. Immediately, he became the darling of local journalists, who pressed him for quotes and sound bites. This media exposure unfairly set Lawson up as the instigator of the movement, and, consequently, made him a target for the vitriol of the *Nashville Banner* and its segregationist publisher, Jimmy Stahlman, a dominant member of the Vanderbilt Board of Trust.

Chancellor Harvie Branscomb was now juggling a sizzling time bomb. On the one hand, he was aware that the rest of the country was moving towards integration and he knew that in order for Vanderbilt to qualify for grants and to be taken seriously as a national research university, it would have to follow suit. Branscomb had set up a delib-erate, calculated approach for that to happen. The civil rights movement in general and Vanderbilt Divinity student James Lawson in particular were messing up the whole program. The university's fragile reputation was on the line.

Branscomb first tried to work through Divinity Dean Robert Nelson, sending him as the intermediary to make Lawson aware of a new policy in the student handbook forbidding students to "participate in disorderly assemblies, or assemblies likely to lead to disorder." The rule had recently been added as an attempt to squelch panty raids.[6] Lawson, however, was unapologetic and unwilling to recant his statements to the mayor.

Branscomb then made what he would later admit was a tactical error. The Executive Committee of the Board of Trust had a scheduled meeting for March 3, and the Chancellor decided to bring the Lawson incident before the board. James Stahlman had hit pay dirt. He swore and ranted and wielded his power on the board. By unanimous decision, the committee voted to have Lawson either withdraw from the university or face expulsion. Lawson chose to be expelled.

With the Executive Committee empowered to call the shots, Branscomb had lost control of the situation. Upon hearing the news of Lawson's expulsion, members of the Divinity School faculty remonstrated and demanded that Lawson, who was an exemplary student, either be reinstated or they would resign. The dispute hit the national wires as students and faculty from other departments joined in campus protest marches, holding placards that read: "Academic Freedom Stifled" and "Expulsion Unfair."

In the midst of the bedlam came an interesting turn of events in the medical school. Several faculty members approached Christie insisting that they, too, would resign unless the affair was settled in Lawson's favor. Christie answered that, in that case, he'd have to accept their resignations. Randy Batson was similarly approached and gave the same response. These two men had been responsible twelve years earlier for defiantly integrating the pediatric ward, but now they refused to side with Lawson or any of the other protesters.

Sarah Sell had an office across from Amos Christie, whose office was located on the way to the Medical School dean's. Many who entered the dean's office had to first pass by Christie. The pediatric chief watched droves of agitated faculty members and trustees tramping by day after day.

Sell said, "He told me that for the good of the university . . . his money was on the Chancellor. Dr. Christie said that whatever power he had he was going to swing it with Branscomb."[7]

Amos Christie had several rationales for throwing his lot with the administration. First, although he was exceedingly liberal-minded for his day and age, and personally had no problem with integration, he was uncomfortable with the concept of civil disobedience. He believed in the hierarchy of power and that pathways to change should start at the top. Second, Chancellor Branscomb had stood behind Christie a decade earlier when Dean Goodpasture proposed to convert the medical school into a research institute. Christie believed that Branscomb was now in need of similar support.

Explained Robert Merrill, "Dr. Christie and loyalty were synonymous."

Finally, Christie harbored an acute fear that unless the dissidents were quashed, or at least ignored, and if racial issues were allowed to fester and boil, Vanderbilt University would eventually crumble. He and other long-term faculty members were still smarting from the financial crises of previous years. He was convinced that Vanderbilt, his beloved institution, was in real danger of falling into irreparable disarray.

Christie later wrote of the experience:

> It was possible for several of us to demonstrate what I think might have been leadership, and to show . . . the Chancellor that the Medical School was not going to fold, even if we lost these faculty members. This forced many of us to realize that the University was first and foremost. It would be here long after we were gone and that some of the issues brought up by the Lawson incident were secondary to the stability of the University.[8]

By the end of June 1960, the Lawson incident was over. The downtown lunch counters opened to black citizens. Branscomb reinstated any faculty members who chose to withdraw their resignations, firmly informing angry trustees that this was a matter for the administration to decide and not the board. By that time, said historian Ridley Wills, "Branscomb regretted ever having taken the Lawson decision to the board. He should have just left it to the school."[9]

James Lawson was given the opportunity to finish his degree at Vanderbilt Divinity School but opted instead to accept an offer of matriculation by Boston University. In 1962, Vanderbilt University implemented a policy for integrating the student body, although it would be two years before black students began enrolling. And in

1967, Dr. James Carter, a pediatrician and nutritionist, was appointed as assistant professor in the Vanderbilt Pediatrics Department, the Medical Center's first full-time African American faculty member. Amos Christie was always proud of that fact.[10]

The lunch counter sit-ins and the Lawson incident exposed a side of Nashville that was excruciating to those who loved the city and had been proud of its composure and unity during prior natural disasters and social upheaval. They watched in horror as black students from institutions that brought honor to the city faced abuse. Nashvillians knew that the Tennessee State University women's track team led by Wilma Rudolph was setting Olympic records and bringing home gold medals. They had likewise spent a century boasting about the prestige engendered by the famed a cappella group, the Fisk Jubilee Singers. Former Junior League President Joanne Bailey said, "[The Fisk Jubilee Singers] were one reason we were known as the Athens of the South."[11]

White citizens were also appalled that hoodlums were representing them in the national media. Even if they weren't wholeheartedly in favor of racial integration, they were adamantly opposed to the hooliganism that had been taking place. First, the Hattie Cotton Elementary School had been bombed; then the Jewish Community Center; and during the sit-ins, the home of black attorney Z. Alexander Looby was dynamited, although he survived unhurt. Looby was an exemplary citizen and community leader and was admired by blacks and whites alike. To top that off, hatemongers continued to attack black students. Nashvillians were fed up with divisiveness and nastiness. They wanted the outside world to know that they were striving every day to address these problems. Still, they were wary of haste.

"I think Nashville has always worked *gradually* towards change," said native Nashvillian and former Junior League President Frances Jackson.[12]

The aftershocks from the racial incidents of 1960 oozed into every pore and fissure in the veneer of the community. At the headquarters of the Junior League, members of the League's Executive Committee began to take stock of their own policies—and they were shaken by what they saw. For nearly forty years, they had been denying access to health care to some of the most vulnerable among them in Middle Tennessee—black children. Although these children were allowed into the clinics at the Junior League Home, they could not be admitted as residents.

Mary Lee Manier was the president of the Junior League in Nashville during that period, and she embarked into some fairly painful soul-searching. "You can't believe how awful things were in terms of racial discrimination," she said, "and we accepted it. It was unbelievable."[13]

Manier called a meeting of the Executive Committee of the Junior League and proposed that since they were already broadening the definition of the crippled child, they should expand it to include black children as well. Fortunately, the Executive Committee was made up of some of the most progressive members in the League and they unanimously approved the measure. It also helped that the staff of nurses and therapists were strongly in favor of admitting black patients.[14] Now, they had to get the approval of the membership at large— which would not be nearly as easy. Some Junior League members were, in fact, related or married to men whose downtown businesses were affected by the protesters.

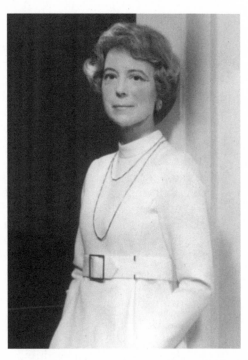

In 1958, the League had investigated the possibility of allowing black patients to be admitted to the Home, citing the following reasons in its report: "There [were] no

During her tenure as president of the Junior League of Nashville, Mary Lee Manier led the charge to integrate the Home and to support the opening of a community children's hospital.

facilities for the convalescent care of Negro children in this section of the state . . ." and "Admitting Negro children to the Home would cause no real problems—none have been experienced at Vanderbilt Hospital where the pediatric service is no longer segregated."[15]

After consideration, the proposal was rejected because Meharry was trying to institute an orthopedic program and would need the children as teaching material, but also for reasons attributed to "changing times":

a) The effect of integration on the parents of patients in the Home and on the Staff of the Home was questioned.
b) The placing of a negro [sic] orthopedic surgeon on the Medical Staff of the Junior League Home for Crippled Children caused concern among some of the physicians on the Staff.

The committee decided that the Junior League's interests would be better served by giving financial assistance to the Meharry orthopedic program or by raising funds for a convalescent home near Meharry. The report concluded with this action:

Since the Home Board has been advised by the majority of the Medical Staff at the Home, by the majority of the pediatricians present at the meeting held with the Nashville Pediatric Society and by the majority of the orthopedic and plastic surgeons present at the meeting held with them, that such a move would be detrimental to the orthopedic teaching program at Meharry Medical School, it was moved that no further consideration be given at this time to the admission of negro [sic] patients.[16]

In the intervening two years, attitudes toward this subject changed dramatically. The Executive Committee, made up of young women, presented their proposal for integration to the membership, comprised of ladies of all ages. Some were fine with the idea. Others, particularly some of the sustaining members, were irate. Certain members threatened to quit the Junior League.

Mary Lee Manier and the committee expected a backlash. "But we still knew it was the right thing to do," she said. "I think just about everybody thought it was right for those little children to have care."

As far as she recalled, nobody quit the League in the end. She did have to speak individually to some concerned members. One woman approached her and said that she didn't want her daughter, who was a provisional, working with black children at the Home. At that time, volunteering at the Home was a requirement for provisional members. Manier explained that the daughter wasn't required to have contact with the children, but could instead volunteer in some other way, such as filing papers or answering phones in the office. As it turned out, the daughter actually approved of the measure and had no desire to be stuck in an office when she could be helping with children instead.

Ultimately, integration of the Home proceeded fairly rapidly and without commotion. In December 1960, Home Board Chair Mary Cooper Beazley, wife of pediatrician Luther Beazley, oversaw the admission of three black children to the Home. By then, members had gotten used to the idea, and the change happened with remarkably little fallout.[17]

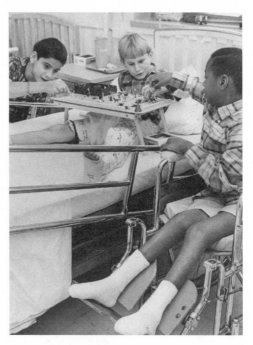

Following the sit-ins at the downtown lunch counters, the Junior League of Nashville reexamined its policies and integrated its Home for Crippled Children. Photo by J. T. Phillips.

The Junior League administration had deftly overcome a number of obstacles. It had convinced the membership to go along with integration. Having sought the advice of Joe Greathouse, Associate Director of Vanderbilt University Hospital, about how Vanderbilt Pediatrics had managed to maintain an integrated unit with little outside argument, they discovered that Vanderbilt had heard very few complaints from parents about the practice of placing white and black patients in the same room. "The majority of these complaints," Greathouse told them, "have been concerned with the necessity of white and Negro parents standing side by side to view infants in the nursery, whose cribs are placed without regard to race."[18]

Ultimately, patients' families at the Home for Crippled Children were far more accommodating and less disturbed by the new policy than expected. And Meharry, consequently, had some place for its pediatric patients to convalesce. Only one problem

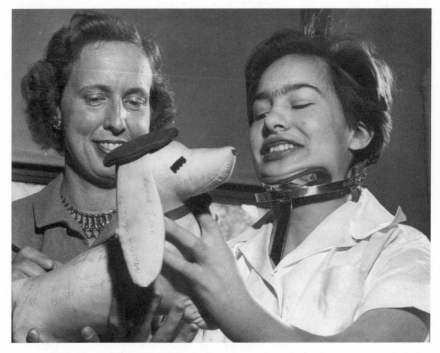

In 1960, Home Board Chair Mary Cooper Beazley, at left with a patient, oversaw the integration of the Junior League Home for Crippled Children, which took place without incident or commotion.

remained—convincing any local pediatricians and dentists, who donated their time to see patients at the Home but who had policies against treating black children, to continue volunteering.

League members knew it would require finesse to get these crucial participants to buy into their plans. Luckily, finesse was their forte. They sent out letters to their health care providers explaining all the changes in the admission requirements, including that they were now raising the maximum age of white children to fifteen, accepting children with any number of disabilities who might benefit from convalescent care, and admitting to the Home "Negro children up to twelve years of age only because of our connection with the city school system."

The letter said that providers could contact the Home administrator if they had any questions about the new admission requirements. It concluded with, "Let me thank you again for your continued cooperation."[19]

In other words, the Junior League simply made the issue nonnegotiable. To continue operation, they would have to comply with the school system, and the schools were in the process of integrating. Ironically, the Junior League Home integrated without a hitch long before those in charge of the Nashville public school system figured out how to do so.

The leadership of the Junior League of Nashville had one more motivation for integrating the Home. A group of physicians and businessmen had approached them and asked for their support in an effort to build a children's hospital. Mary Lee Manier and her cohorts understood that if they were going to back such a project, it would have to serve all members of the community—all races and all socioeconomic classes. The League Home needed to be already assisting those populations if they were to make a valid argument.

Little did they know in 1960 that the campaign for a children's hospital would prove to be the lengthiest, most vicious battle they ever faced.

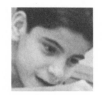

Jousting for Power and Control | 9

"They are kicking the crutch out from under the crippled child!"

—Saying by Junior League members about those who would not support a children's hospital in Nashville

Dr. George Holcomb would hardly strike anyone as a rabble-rouser. Soft-spoken and deferential, he had graduated from Vanderbilt Medical School, spent a three-year residency in adult surgery, and then transferred for an additional three years into a residency program at Boston Children's Hospital. At the end of his training, he was drafted into the Korean War and stationed in Osaka, Japan. Upon completing his military obligations, Holcomb returned to Nashville and opened up a private surgical practice where he saw both adult and pediatric patients—typical of the way nearly all the local surgeons ran their practices. Yet, unlike them, when he visited his young patients on the pediatric wards of the local hospitals, he was dissatisfied. He kept thinking about his experience in Boston at a hospital set up exclusively for children, where nurses, social workers, and cleaning crew were all geared to address the specific needs of youngsters.

In Nashville's hospitals, he encountered nurses who didn't even like children assigned to pediatric rotations. Other staff members were fond enough of children, but had no interest in dealing with parents. Lab tests, hospital equipment, beds, chairs—everything in the local hospitals being used for and by children had been originally intended for grown-ups. He and his fellow surgeons routinely had to take surgical instruments designed for adults and try to adapt them for tiny bodies. During this early stage of his career, an inspiration came to him—a vision that would spawn an astonishingly long and persistent crusade. Nashville, Holcomb thought, had a crucial need for a children's hospital. Once he became certain of this, he felt he had to convince the residents of the city, area health care officials, and the leaders of the four major hospitals—Vanderbilt, Meharry, Baptist, and St. Thomas—of the value of constructing such a building.[1]

Holcomb was not proposing a revolutionary idea. The first children's hospital in the English-speaking world had opened up in London in 1852, with the support of novelist Charles Dickens, who helped raise money for it by giving readings from *A Christmas Carol*.[2] Three years later, the Children's Hospital of Philadelphia, the first on American soil, opened under the guidance of Dr. Francis Lewis West, who had paid a visit to the London facility. In that age of American medicine, most sick children and infants were treated at home to avoid cross-infections they picked up at adult hospitals. West believed that academic medicine and specialized care would move forward much more efficiently if young patients were admitted to a dedicated pediatric facility rather than placing them on a pediatric ward in an institution that also treated sick adults.[3] By 1883, ten

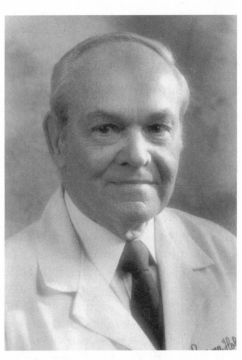

Pediatric surgeon Dr. George Holcomb spent over twenty-five years lobbying for Nashville to build a children's hospital.

children's hospitals were operating in North America, with most of them concentrated in the Northeast and three in larger cities of the Midwest.[4]

By the 1950s, when Holcomb opened his practice, dozens of children's hospitals had sprung up across the nation, and they tended to have a common legacy. Usually, a group of strong-willed, civic-minded women determined the need for such a facility, purchased a local home or office building, and paid to have it converted into a small children's hospital that served only a few patients at a time. Also by mid-century, the national Shriners organization was sponsoring numerous children's hospitals for burn victims and children with orthopedic problems. As the century progressed, however, the push for children's hospitals began to arise from local surgeons rather than pediatricians.

After the retirement of Barney Brooks, Dr. H. William Scott Jr. took over as chairman of surgery at Vanderbilt. Scott had trained in general pediatric surgery at Boston Children's Hospital and later gained extensive experience in pediatric heart surgery while a resident at Johns Hopkins. As leader of the Vanderbilt surgery department, he opened up a rotation for house staff known as pediatric surgery, the only one of its kind in the country at that time.

That residency rotation lured James O'Neill to Vanderbilt. O'Neill later wrote of Scott:

> While he was always a general surgeon, he had a long-standing interest and devotion to pediatric surgery, and he did it very well, at least by the standards of that time. When I first arrived on the scene as an intern in 1959, he was really the pediatric surgeon at Vanderbilt. Since pediatrics was such a small service, it was hard for anyone to devote their energies entirely to pediatric surgery then.[5]

The same year that Scott arrived in Nashville, Dr. William Hillman was appointed assistant professor of orthopedic surgery at Vanderbilt. Hillman became renowned for his work with children born with handicaps, birth defects, scoliosis, and cerebral palsy. Hillman "possessed an enormous capacity for work"[6] and researched a wide range of physiological processes that led to pediatric bone and joint disease. In the past, the role of doctors had been to help make life more bearable for children with congenital problems. By the 1960s, however, surgeons like Scott, Hillman, O'Neill, and Holcomb—physicians with brave new energy and expertise—were filtering into Nashville. They were eager to give surgical solutions a try, to test out pioneering operations that were unheard of only a few years earlier. They knew that the ideal environment for engaging in these daring and novel approaches would be a children's hospital.[7]

Holcomb was so sure of the value of this mission that he was willing to stand up to the existing regime and plead his case. Since there were no pediatric surgeons in that era, and since general surgeons had no desire to relinquish their pediatric cases, Holcomb would have to win the support for a children's hospital from area pediatricians. He first sought the advice of his old mentor, Amos Christie, who at that time wielded an enormous amount of power in the field. Christie had reigned as the chairman of pediatrics for over fifteen years by then and had concrete ideas about what was required for a quality system of pediatric care. A children's hospital, he informed Holcomb, definitely didn't fit into his plans or into his budget—although he was much more tight-lipped about the latter issue. His concerns were legitimate. Freestanding children's hospitals were (and are) notoriously costly to run, a painful truth that cities across America were starting to discover.

Christie wrote in his memoir:

> I vigorously opposed the projection of this hospital as a citizen with some health facility planning knowledge.
> I did not think it would hurt Vanderbilt immediately, but the economy of a freestanding hospital is so tenuous that it would be just a question of time until having built an expensive hospital with many duplications of services, they would get in trouble staffing and financing it. There would inevitably be a problem of filling the beds with patients that somebody else would have to pay for. . . .[8]

The pediatric chief's curt dismissal of the proposal cut Holcomb to the core. Interestingly, neither man allowed this gaping disagreement to affect their professional relationship. Christie still held the young surgeon in high regard and continued to refer patients to him and help him build up his budding surgical practice. In turn, Holcomb retired for a while to the wings. But he wasn't giving up. In fact, he was gathering information.

By the time he'd been in practice for five years and had the raw numbers in front of him, Holcomb was more resolute than ever, believing that Nashville was behind the times in its delivery of health care and treatment of children. He'd run his data upside down and sideways, and every calculation indicated that the city had a current shortage of over 150 pediatric beds. That number was only going to increase with each coming year, until by 1970 Nashville's hospitals would be short 235 beds, presenting a genuine crisis in the health care of its youngest citizens.[9]

Holcomb realized he was going to have to pull together a community coalition if he had any chance of winning support from Vanderbilt. One of the first groups he called upon was the Junior League. Ever since the League's merger with the Council of Jewish Women's Convalescent Home, problems at the Home had become more worrisome. The house on White Avenue was aging and in need of extensive repairs. The children admitted as residents were much sicker than the orthopedic patients who once exclusively convalesced there. Although Christie was sending his house staff and faculty to the Home to attend to patients with acute and chronic medical problems, League members often received phone calls in the middle of the day or night asking them to transport medically distressed children to the emergency rooms of Vanderbilt and Nashville General Hospitals.

In 1961, eleven-year-old Beth Odle stayed as an inpatient at the Junior League Home for three months while her surgeon, Dr. Eugene Regen, readied her for an operation to correct a severe curvature of the spine. Beth was from Wartrace, Tennessee, about sixty miles southeast of Nashville. She had never been away from home before and never spent time apart from her mother. Terrified when she first arrived, and surrounded by sick children, she prayed every night that she wouldn't die there. Although she had to remain in traction for several hours each day, the rest of the time she was up and about. Since she was mobile, she soon befriended other kids at the Home.

Odle recalled:

> Some children had to go through lots of operations and then come back to the Home to recover.
> I mostly remember the kids with [hydrocephalus].[10] Their heads were so huge they could hardly sit up. Other kids had massive body casts that covered their entire bodies. Their legs were spread apart with a bar between them and a hole cut out so they could go to the bathroom.[11]

The census of the Home had dramatically changed. League members were often caring for chronically ill children, some of whom would not survive. They found themselves in uncharted territory, explaining to youngsters at the Home about fatal diseases, abandonment, and death. Nothing in their provisional training courses had prepared them for that.

In addition, because the Home had opened its admissions to include nonindigent children, the Junior League had to find a way to accept insurance payments and partial payments. Given its current status, the Home could not meet the labyrinth of regulatory criteria demanded by insurance companies. Then again, members could hardly justify drawing money from the Trust Fund to pay for children whose parents were insured and capable of making payments. As a Band-Aid solution, they asked families with insurance to make a donation to the Home to defray the cost of caring for their children.

Junior League President Mary Lee Manier met with her executive committee in a touchy, gut-wrenching debate. The committee acceded that the time had come to turn the operation of the Home for Crippled Children over to an outside agency. They would devote money in the Trust towards a smooth transition.

Around this same time, George Holcomb approached the League and asked for its support in the construction of a freestanding regional children's hospital. The women thought their prayers had been answered. Perhaps they'd found their redeemer. They could simply move the children from the Home onto a special convalescent ward of the new hospital. Their children would be tended by nurses and staff well trained in the care of the severely ill, with emergency facilities practically on their doorstep. In spite of several obvious pitfalls, the executive committee decided that, much like its determination to integrate the Home, this was simply the right thing to do. Now all they needed was a hospital.

Having won the cooperation of the Junior League leadership, Holcomb then spoke to the Al Menah Shriners. They agreed to transfer the proceeds of the lucrative Palm Sunday Paper Sale to the new hospital, which ensured a substantial annual income for the venture. With diligence and diplomacy, the surgeon methodically approached and appealed to the scions of Nashville's social and political powers. Business leaders flocked to the project. Entrepreneur Jack Massey stepped up as fund chairman. Bill Weaver, president of National Life, joined the fray.

Thrilled by the possibilities, local pediatricians such as Ethel Walker, Tommy Zerfoss, Luther Beazley, and William Vaughn, among others, offered their assistance by calling upon local organizations for support. The Council of Jewish Women, the Nashville Academy of

Medicine, the Tennessee Orthopaedic Society, and the Nashville Pediatric Society came on board. Child psychiatrists were excited about having a hospital where they could admit children with less serious emotional illnesses, since Vanderbilt was building a unit that would be restricted to the severely emotionally disturbed.[12]

Holcomb made his appeal to group after group, stating:

> First and foremost is the consideration of the children of this community: yours and mine. Children from all levels of social and economic groups alike. It is hoped that this will not be just a private hospital nor one for the so-called indigent persons. It is the plan to provide for both. There are people who desire their children to have the best accommodations available and are financially capable for the remuneration for the expense. These people have a right to such. There are those who have the same desire for their children but cannot afford the additional expense. These people have the right to have decent, well lighted, airy, pleasant surroundings while their children are ill. To provide for both extremes and the middle is the desire, goal and aims of this children's hospital.[13]

Naturally, as the momentum and excitement began to escalate, so did the local politics. Baptist Hospital began to show interest, since a children's hospital would free up adult beds in its main hospital. Sister Henrietta Neuhoff of St. Thomas Hospital became a cautious advocate as well. St. Thomas had lost its pediatric accreditation a few years earlier because it lacked the capacity to educate and train interns and nurses for the service. As a result, surgeons practicing at St. Thomas had to admit their pediatric patients to adult wards, since there was no medical pediatrics unit on site.[14] Sensing the chance to regain a foothold in pediatrics, St. Thomas bought into the idea.

In addition, Public Health Director John Lentz became a drum major for the project, proclaiming that he would send all of the pediatric patients currently seen at Nashville General to the new community hospital. This announcement left Amos Christie dumbfounded. For years, Vanderbilt had been responsible for the pediatric service at Nashville General Hospital, where his residents gained valuable experience while rounding there. The transfer of those patients to a community facility would demolish a major source of Vanderbilt's pediatric teaching material. To protect his house staff, Christie realized he'd have to go on the offensive.

In the swirl of the fracas, Chancellor Harvie Branscomb became pinned in a corner. The administrators at Baptist, St. Thomas, and Nashville General were uniting into a voting bloc, leaving Vanderbilt and Meharry, the other teaching medical school in town, isolated and vulnerable. Branscomb felt obligated to appease his medical faculty, who opposed the plan, while also mollifying members of his Board of Trust, some of whom would benefit personally and professionally by the construction of a children's hospital in town. Meanwhile, board members, such as Hank Ingram, were being squeezed by their wives to get an honest answer out of Vanderbilt about whether or not the institution was truly interested in taking over the Home for Crippled Children. Eventually, Hortense Ingram had attended one emotional League meeting too many. Exasperated, she announced to the membership that it was time to cut to the chase. "I'm going to go talk to the Chancellor!" she declared.[15]

Her daughter Alice Hooker said, "She got tired of Vanderbilt being wishy-washy about wanting to take over [the Home]. So she went marching into the Chancellor's office and said, 'Don't miss this opportunity! It's your responsibility! You'd better get with this program with the Junior League!'"[16]

Forced into mediation, Branscomb delivered an olive branch to the Junior League in the form of a proposal:

> Vanderbilt University is aware of the great service that the Junior League has rendered to Nashville, and wishes to cooperate in every possible way with future developments. Meetings have been held by the Hospital Committee of the Board of Trust and by various faculty groups, and the following proposals are made to the Junior League for their consideration.
>
> (1) If it is the decision of the Junior League to construct a new Home for Crippled Children to provide convalescent care, Vanderbilt University will make available without cost land adjacent to the University Hospital.
>
> (2) If the Junior League decides that it wishes to develop an institution for children more extensive than a convalescent home then Vanderbilt University will:
>
> (a) Make land available, without cost, adjacent to the Vanderbilt Hospital, and
>
> (b) As the sponsors of the hospital may wish, take part in discussions aimed at merging the interests of the Junior League's present program for convalescent care, the

responsibilities of the University including its house
staff program, and the needs of the private practitioners into a cooperative entity for the benefit of the
whole community.[17]

Essentially, Branscomb was willing to donate land for the building,
with the understanding that the new facility would maintain the stamp
of Vanderbilt. Although various factions wanted Vanderbilt to participate in the children's hospital, many of them had no desire for the
University to reign supreme over it. In response, Baptist Hospital
geared up for a jousting match. Administrators at Baptist issued a
"Statement of Belief As Concerns A Children's Hospital for Nashville,"
in which they stated their desire for a "separate and distinct complete
hospital for the total care of children in the community," operating
under its own bylaws and constitution. To that end, Baptist offered to
donate unused land it owned in its hospital center for the building, with
the notation that "Baptist Hospital is not interested in making a profit
on any of its unused property for this most worthwhile project."[18]

These offers and counteroffers of land for the proposed children's
hospital were less an embarrassment of riches and generosity than a
crafty game of keep-away among the major players.

Compelled to get involved, the Chamber of Commerce called for
a feasibility study to see if Nashville actually had as great a need as
advocates claimed. The Chamber hired a nationally known hospital
consultant, Dr. W. T. Sanger of Sanger-Beale Associates, to evaluate
whether the timing was right for such an undertaking. Sanger's initial
report, much to the relief of the Vanderbilt administration, stated that
"a new freestanding children's hospital is not indicated."[19]

Surprisingly, the Sanger report did little to stem the enthusiasm
of the hospital's proponents. They continued their pursuits and
converted more and more believers—and stoked the ire of disbelievers.
During the summer of 1961, the clamor regarding the children's
hospital reached a fever pitch. In an attempt to circumvent Christie,
members of the Junior League and other hospital proponents had
been meeting with Vanderbilt officials without including the pediatric
chief in their discussions. Christie was aware these meetings were
taking place and also knew that he was being bypassed by the officials
of the medical school and hospital administration.[20]

According to historian Paul Conkin, this was a period of great
internal turmoil among the Vanderbilt medical faculty. Dean

Goodpasture's successor, John Youmans, had resigned after a short
tenure and Dr. John W. Patterson had taken over. In 1959, Patterson
was dubbed with the new title of vice chancellor for medical affairs.
"Patterson administered efficiently. He ruled arbitrarily," Conkin
said. By 1961, Patterson had so alienated the older, venerated faculty
members that they grouped together to call for his ouster, accusing
him of making irresponsible, dictatorial, "high-handed decisions"
without consulting them. During one clash, Christie blatantly defied
Patterson's orders. Both men took their case to Branscomb, who
stood by his chairman and fired the vice chancellor. Branscomb then
named Randy Batson, Christie's gentle-spirited, collegial protégé, as
Patterson's replacement.[21]

With Batson in place, the in-house acrimony quickly receded.
Therefore, the political hot potato that had been tossed both
within the walls of Vanderbilt University, as well as back and forth
between the Medical School and the community, landed back in the
palms of the proponents of the children's hospital. Christie had
repeatedly expressed concern that a freestanding community children's
hospital would directly compete with Vanderbilt pediatrics. Unless
the facility belonged to Vanderbilt, he could not agree to participate.
Holcomb and company decided to offer Christie the golden ring.
Although the new hospital would be governed by an outside board
of trustees consisting of community members—such as delegates
from the Junior League; members of the Chamber of Commerce
and business and industry; and physicians representing pediatrics,
orthopedics, surgery, and psychiatry—they would appoint Amos
Christie as medical director. Surely, they thought, he would jump at
the chance to take the helm of this elite assembly. Instead, Christie
recoiled at their offer. The last thing he wanted was to be in charge
of such a risky enterprise.

Holcomb explained, "He was saying that to run a university
organization or department, he had to be in complete control. He
didn't want to take a vote in a board meeting and lose by two votes on
what to do."[22]

The ladies of the Junior League were shocked and infuriated by
Christie's response and by Vanderbilt's reluctance to intervene. They
couldn't fathom why anybody would be opposed to a children's
hospital. Grousing among themselves, Leaguers charged that those
who did not support the new children's hospital were, "kicking the
crutch out from under the crippled child!"[23]

According to James O'Neill, there was more to Christie's aversion than a demand for authority. "Dr. Christie didn't know how to behave with a big community group," O'Neill said.

> Despite the fact that he was a strong personality, he was actually shy around community leaders. Amos Christie was interested in bacteriology and histoplasmosis and obscure things that happened to children, and he'd used them to teach. This kind of entrepreneurial development was foreign to him . . . Entrepreneurs would scare him to death.[24]

In any case, Christie's refusal to serve as medical director delivered a harsh blow to a committee working hard to be fair and open-minded. In July of 1961, Dr. Addison Scoville, who had trained under Christie and was also a member of the Health and Hospitals Committee of the Chamber of Commerce, asked his old mentor for a meeting to discuss the children's hospital controversy. In the heading of his report of that meeting, Scoville wrote, "Circumstances: This discussion was done on an individual personal basis as an expression of respect of a former house officer to the chief of service."[25] All over town, pediatricians were feeling equally torn about facing down their beloved mentor. Here stood two synods of honorable people confronting each other over a common humanitarian calling, but failing to see eye-to-eye.

Christie told Scoville that he understood that the proponents had the best interest of the community's children in mind, but he warned that their ill-conceived venture would impair the teaching abilities at Vanderbilt, Meharry, and Nashville General Hospitals. Because Vanderbilt's credentialing committee was imposing stricter guidelines, he could not guarantee that physicians at the new hospital could also obtain a university appointment. He also added that if the hospital were seen to be in conflict with Vanderbilt, he would withdraw the privileges of visiting staff with current appointments. Christie added that his tenure would be up in about seven more years, when he planned to retire, and that he could not be responsible for Vanderbilt's future beyond that.[26] In other words, the only carrot he dangled before Scoville was "maybe you should try again later."

That same week, George Holcomb sent Christie a letter to inform him of the committee's progress.

As a former student and recently as a medical colleague, I have always had the highest respect and admiration for you and always will. I shall be grateful forever for your encouragement and personal support, which you gave me when I returned to Nashville. For these reasons, I want you to be aware of my motives and interest in the proposed Nashville Children's Hospital. I don't envision this hospital competing with your program at all. . . .[27]

Christie answered Holcomb's letter the next day:

. . . I congratulate you on your effort. I am impressed by the prodigious amount of work which has gone into preparation of such a plan as you envision . . . I feel caught in a trap. My responsibility is obvious. It will always be my hope that with the possible development of a children's hospital in Nashville ways can be found for not dividing us into two competitive groups or camps.[28]

Christie went on to describe the new clinical building that Vanderbilt was constructing, including plans to close the polio unit and use those beds for a "top-flight children's surgical unit of approximately 30 beds," and to add 10 beds for private pediatric patients, as well as to enlarge the nursery.[29]

". . . I realize fully the limitations which even this advance might place on you," he continued. " . . . As you know, this will give us a 125 to 135 bed children's hospital-within-a-hospital. . . ."[30]

Earlier, Vanderbilt department heads sent Randy Batson on a fact-finding tour that included a trip to California. Batson returned to Vanderbilt with the notion that the new west wing of the hospital should be constructed as an in-the-round facility. On each floor, nursing and staff services would occupy the center space with patient rooms extending like spokes from the central axis. Although Christie was a student of the old school, the idea of a circular pediatric ward pleased him.

In mid-July, Dr. Paul Morrissey Jr., chairman of the Health and Hospitals Committee of the Chamber of Commerce, called a discreet meeting of interested parties to again review the efficacy of building a children's hospital. He also asked W. T. Sanger, the consultant, to return to Nashville to conduct a follow-up survey about the need for such a facility, given the changes that had taken place during the past year.

The discretion was short-lived. On July 26, 1961, reporter Jack Setters launched a series of articles in the *Nashville Banner* casting aspersions on the concept of a community children's hospital. "Vanderbilt Children's Hospital Is Already Under Construction," blasted one headline. "Need For Another Facility Being Questioned By Many." The story stated that when Vanderbilt Hospital's circular west wing was completed, it would be "larger than most metropolitan pediatrics hospitals in the nation," and that erecting a second facility in town would "necessitate the duplication of existing facilities at an enormous cost." Christie touted the benefit of having a medical school and hospital under the same roof. And to address another gnawing issue, he declared that Vanderbilt's Pediatrics Department and the expanded "children's hospital-within-a-hospital" would be open to all Nashville pediatricians. Patient rooms would be state-of-the-art, equipped with closed circuit television sets and adjacent to a large playroom.[31]

The next day, Setters ran a story stating that city finance director Joe Torrence was withdrawing John Lentz's promise to move the pediatric patients at Nashville General to the planned community hospital. He cited the admirable job that Vanderbilt was doing in running Nashville General's twenty-nine-bed pediatrics department. Torrence expressed concern about the cost of constructing the new facility, which had bloomed from an estimated $2 million to $5 million. He added that as far as he knew, plans for the community project were only in the "embryonic stage."[32]

By September, Sanger had returned to a conference in Nashville where he issued his second report after reevaluating the climate. While acknowledging the acute shortage of pediatric beds in town, he also warned constituents against being "too hasty" to build a children's hospital.

"It's sort of like marriage," Sanger stated, "except that there is no Reno to turn to if it fails."[33]

He told attendees that this ambitious project would have to be supported by tax monies and at least one major private fund-raising campaign. He explained that a good many of the nation's children's hospitals were in financial trouble and that of the forty-seven such hospitals operating in the United States, thirty-four were connected to medical schools. Sanger insinuated that if their plans had any chance of reaching fruition, Vanderbilt had to fit into the equation. He then directed attention to the Junior League Home for Crippled

Children, which by that time was internationally applauded for its groundbreaking approach to convalescent care. Nevertheless, the League was planning to turn over the building on White Avenue to the state of Tennessee the following year.

Joanne Bailey represented the Junior League at the Sanger conference. She told those in attendance that the League was in no hurry to invest in the construction of a children's hospital until all the potential problems had been explored. She added that the League membership had not yet voted on whether or not to endorse the project. Ethel Walker then stepped up to explain that, as both a League member and a pediatrician, she wanted to make it known that the convalescing children presently residing at the Home would "not be thrust out into the snow" even though the Home was closing.[34]

By October, Holcomb realized that the wheels were coming off his plans for a children's hospital. The *Banner* ran an eloquent, poetic

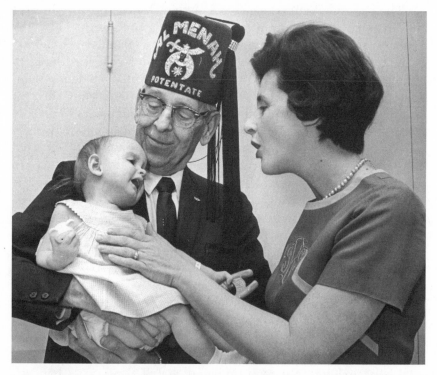

Joanne Bailey (pictured with Potentate Jimmy White) represented the interests of the Junior League of Nashville at the 1961 citywide conference about the feasibility of building a children's hospital in Nashville.

editorial entitled, "Sanger Warns Against Leap In The Dark." In it, the paper's editors agreed with Sanger's suggestion that the wisest approach for the city would be to add a pediatric wing to an existing general hospital (which, appropriately enough, Vanderbilt was already in the process of doing). The editorial ended with the line: "His advice surely isn't given in vain; it must be followed."[35]

A few days later, George Holcomb sent another letter to Dr. Addison Scoville. Holcomb attempted to clarify the proponents' position and to reiterate the need for more beds, "particularly for private patients requiring surgical and medical treatment." He was prepared to give up on capturing the indigent portion of the population if necessary. If need be, the hospital proponents would go it alone without Vanderbilt's endorsement. He wrote:

> I am convinced that having affiliation with the Medical School would improve the teaching program in the Children's Hospital and at Vanderbilt as well. However, if this affiliation is denied by the Medical School, I do not think for a moment that an independent children's hospital would collapse for lack of this affiliation . . . [It] appears unwise to allow any one medical institution to dominate completely any one aspect of patient care to the disadvantage of the others.
>
>   . . . [If] Vanderbilt decides to participate, then we would be most happy. If they do not, then we feel strongly that the community should support it for the benefit of their children. Certainly it should not be stifled by selfish interests emanating from sources which refuse to cooperate.[36]

Holcomb went on to lament that somebody from the Vanderbilt side had leaked information about the discussions to the press before the project had a chance to be presented to the public, noting that the offending newspaper had "contact with the pediatric department at Vanderbilt. . . ."[37]

Holcomb pleaded:

> I hope that you and your committee will appreciate the urgent need for a decision in this matter, because of the Junior League's position and in order to prevent a worthwhile project from being subjected to unfair and unjust verbal and newspaper propaganda while this decision is delayed.[38]

Proponents decided that their only chance of succeeding was to officially organize. In February 1962, the rival *Tennessean* announced that business magnate Jack C. Massey had been elected chairman of the Executive Board of the proposed 125-bed Nashville Children's Hospital. The group's first informational meeting was held at the Junior League Headquarters, presided over by League President Mary Lee Manier, who was also appointed to the board. George Holcomb spoke about methods for covering projected financial deficits, and Health Director John Lentz, in keeping with his flamboyant style, declared that he "would 'fight to my dying day' for the hospital, and urged the board to 'get the show on the road.'"[39]

Whereupon, the project died a quiet death. Or, more accurately, it slipped into a long, deep coma. The reason, said Holcomb, was that despite their Herculean efforts, Amos Christie still refused to budge. While it seemed that the proponents held all the cards, it was Christie who controlled the single most crucial ingredient—the house staff. He was in charge of the interns and residents responsible for the day-to-day supervision of patients, and he was not, said Robert Merrill, going to relinquish that control to anybody. Christie knew that some-times a hospitalized child required round-the-clock attention. A practicing pediatrician with a waiting room full of kids couldn't spend all day in the hospital tending to one particular sick child. But if the need arose, a resident could.[40]

Without access to residents and to the innovations generated within an academic institution, the community hospital lost its attrac-tion to many private pediatricians. Eric Chazen said, "I decided I was not going to have anything to do with building a children's hospital independent of Vanderbilt, and I was very outspoken about that. I was vocally against it."[41]

In the end, for all the promises about the Round Wing becoming a children's hospital-within-a-hospital, it never actually became one, although part of it was sectioned off for pediatric cases. A large play-room never quite made it into the final phase of design. And Christie did not open up his service to every practicing pediatrician in town. Which did not mean that the Chief was simply making empty prom-ises, but rather that he didn't have a mercantile, business-oriented bone in his body. He was a traditionalist. He enjoyed the field of medicine just the way it was. And he never saw any advantage in taking the kinds of risks that might roil the waters. Sarah Sell said,

"He told me he spent his last ten years [as pediatric chairman] fighting a children's hospital."[42]

Christie later lamented that the battle over the children's hospital had damaged some of the friendships he'd made. "My own relationship to some older members of the Junior League has never been the same," he wrote in his memoir. "Nevertheless, the reasoning was sound."[43]

Little did Christie foresee that at the exact same time that plans for a children's hospital were finally dissipating—when he thought he could finally rest easy—one of his physician-scientists was engaged in groundbreaking experiments at Vanderbilt. Over time, her work would mature and flourish, and, in the greatest of paradoxes, she would eventually break down the barriers of two things her department chairman opposed most—pediatric subspecialties and the need for a hospital specifically devoted to the care of young children. Her contributions would soon take on a life of their own because, ironically, she was not among the local pediatricians who favored building a children's hospital.

Saving the Smallest Ones | 10

"Mildred Stahlman had this garden of respirators in the nursery. The room felt strange, almost surreal. When a sick baby would come in, Millie would come into the hospital with an old cardboard suitcase from the 1930s that was brown with yellow stripes. She kept a cot in the utility room. And she'd move into the baby's room and live in there as long as that baby was sick—sitting on a stool, day and night, monitoring that baby in the respirator."

—Dr. William Altemeier, recalling Dr. Mildred Stahlman's development of the Vanderbilt Neonatology Intensive Care Unit

On August 7, 1963, President John F. Kennedy and First Lady Jacqueline Kennedy rushed their newborn son Patrick Bouvier to Boston Children's Hospital. Born five and half weeks prematurely at a weight of 4 lb. 10.5 oz, the little boy was gasping for breath. Dr. Thomas P. Graham was an intern on the neonatology unit of Boston Children's when the Kennedy baby arrived, followed by an entourage of concerned friends and relatives, including his parents, his uncle Bobby Kennedy, and White House Press Secretary Pierre Salinger.[1] Suffering from hyaline membrane disease, or respiratory distress syndrome,[2] Patrick died two days later.

"Gosh, he was a beautiful little baby," said Graham. "He was just breathing like crazy and we couldn't do anything for him."

Baby Kennedy's obituary in the *New York Times* lamented that the only thing that could be done "for a victim of hyaline membrane disease is to monitor the infant's blood chemistry and try to keep it near normal levels. Thus, the battle for the Kennedy baby was lost

121

only because medical science has not yet advanced far enough to accomplish as quickly as necessary what the body can do by itself in its own time."[3]

Ironically, if little Patrick had been born in Nashville and been brought to Vanderbilt Hospital, he might have had a chance to survive. Beginning in 1961, Vanderbilt's Mildred Stahlman had been experimenting with the use of ventilators to save the lives of premature infants—and she was having success. Ventilation machines, such as iron lungs, had originally been built to help children and adults with polio, but the devices were too powerful to be used on tiny babies. The existing apparati might blow out the lungs of premature infants. Physicians were also dogged by the fear of oxygen toxicity. They knew that giving too much oxygen to babies could make them go blind.[4]

Since their intervention options were unacceptable, the most doctors could do for premature infants was to simply wait and watch them die in their cribs—or celebrate as a few lucky ones pulled through. Physicians usually didn't even attempt a remedy.

Stahlman broke with her American colleagues on this protocol. She was convinced that if physicians could understand the physiological processes that occur in the heart and lungs that allow babies to thrive in utero and continue thriving outside the womb after birth, they could mechanically replicate those conditions for premature infants. Stahlman joined a handful of daring investigators who revolutionized neonatology by giving babies born too early time to mature normally by using ventilators to help them breathe.

From her early years, Mildred Stahlman had charted a course for herself that was unique for a woman of her social standing. She never married; lived a frugal, simple lifestyle; and dedicated herself to the male-dominated field of academic medicine. The daughter of *Banner* newspaper publisher Jimmy Stahlman, she inherited from her father his ferocious temper, fierce sense of loyalty, and keen intellect. By the time she started college, Mildred and her sister Ann[5] had already commissioned and christened a war cruiser, the USS *Nashville*. This ship would have a storied career during the Second World War and was selected to be the flagship that transported General Douglas MacArthur on his renowned triumphant return to the Philippines.[6]

As a young Vanderbilt faculty member trained in cardiology, Stahlman received a small grant from the National Institutes of Health to study hyaline membrane disease. When her $11,000 grant came up for renewal in 1959, she tacked on a colossal $125,000 supplement, asking to also build and furnish a nursery with state-of-the-art equipment, along with an attached laboratory. Stahlman received the grant. In the meantime, she, her colleague Dr. Elliott Newman, and a cadre of pediatric fellows had been experimenting with sheep, monitoring the course of hyaline membrane disease by measuring blood gases in fetal lambs. Stahlman kept her sheep at a friend's farm and would drive them in to Nashville when they were needed for study. In those days, Vanderbilt Medical Center was shaped in cross sections, like two Hs, with a little enclosed square of lawn in the center of the complex. Stahlman used to take her sheep to graze on the grass courtyard before bringing them up to the lab. The best way to get the sheep into the courtyard, however, was by herding them through the pediatric clinic.[7]

"Every once in a while there would be a tremendous stench in the corridor, related to the fact that Millie Stahlman's sheep were kept just

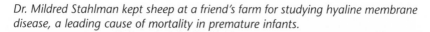

Dr. Mildred Stahlman kept sheep at a friend's farm for studying hyaline membrane disease, a leading cause of mortality in premature infants.

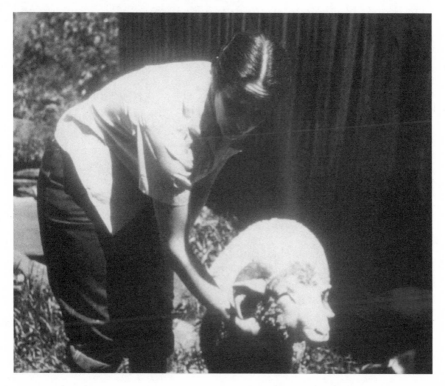

outside the clinic and they would come through on carts during clinic time," said Dr. John Lukens, a pediatric hematologist/oncologist.[8]

Added Ian Burr, "The kids thought it was great, but the parents weren't too thrilled. It was the only way to get to the patch of green."[9]

Within months of opening the newly funded neonatal facility, the first crisis occurred. In October 1961, a senior medical student's baby girl was born at Vanderbilt Hospital two months prematurely. With little hope, the parents and the child's pediatrician granted permission for Stahlman to try to save the baby's life. Stahlman wheeled into the nursery a prototype infant ventilator, a miniature iron lung, which had sat in a basement storage room for years. She hooked it up and then inserted an umbilical venous catheter into the baby girl's left atrium. She sealed the child inside the tank, hoping to keep her alive until her lungs matured to the point where she could breathe on her own. For four days and nights, the doctor and her team monitored the baby's vital signs. Stahlman kept constant vigil, catching fragments of sleep in a foldaway bed she had stashed in the adjacent lab. On the fifth day, the exhausted doctors and nurses realized the little girl was out of the woods and they weaned her off the respirator.[10]

"If that baby hadn't survived, I think I would have quit and done something else," Stahlman said.[11]

As it was, Stahlman was just getting started. By the end of that year, she had created the first modern newborn intensive care unit in the world.[12] She began collecting respirators, positive-pressure pumps, and negative-pressure tanks. With a lack of commercially available equipment, her team developed its own equipment for monitoring tiny bodies. For the next four or five years, Stahlman's nurses and residents had standing orders to call her anytime night or day, weekday or weekend, whenever an infant in respiratory distress was admitted to the hospital.

Bill Altemeier was one of the pediatric residents at that time. He recalled:

> Mildred Stahlman had this garden of respirators in the nursery. The room felt strange, almost surreal. When a sick baby would come in, Millie would come into the hospital with an old cardboard suitcase from the 1930s that was brown with yellow stripes. She kept a cot in the utility room. And she'd move into the baby's room and live in there as long as that baby was sick—sitting on a stool, day and night, monitoring that baby in the respirator.[13]

Stories of Stahlman's expertise, and impatience as a teacher, were legion. She expected of her residents exactly what she demanded of herself—perfection and a passion for what they were doing. A petite, wisp of a woman, she didn't hesitate to terrify her house staff.

Altemeier said, "Residents were scared to go with Millie on rounds. The worst she could do was ignore you, because that meant she didn't even consider you worth her time. So it wasn't so bad when she cussed you out. She'd say, 'Well, GODDAMN!' And you knew you were in trouble. She was a great teacher. She intimidated the hell out of everybody."

Like many others, Altemeier adored her and fought hard to earn her trust. In the end, Stahlman paid him the greatest of compliments by backing him in his bid to become board-certified in neonatology.

Robert Merrill also became one of Stahlman's greatest champions. The friendship was "hard-earned, hard-earned," he said. "She's integrity personified. There's not a false note in her anywhere." Back in his early days as a faculty member, he was part of a group that she would call together to listen to the talks she would present at scientific conferences. She liked to first practice in front of her peers to get their opinions. Merrill recalled sitting in on one such trial run. Although Stahlman had collected groundbreaking data on her experiments with premature infants and respirators, her slides were terrible. They were so packed with numbers that they were hard to read and impossible to assimilate. Unfortunately, everybody in the group was afraid to tell her that.

Finally Merrill spoke up, "It's a great paper, but you're going to have to do something about your slides."

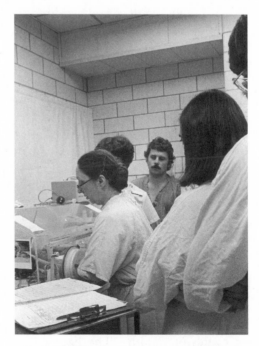

Dr. Mildred Stahlman's nurses and residents had standing orders to call her anytime night or day, whenever an infant in respiratory distress was admitted to the hospital.

"Goddamn!" she barked, "What do you mean?"

"Sorry, Millie, but they just won't do," Merrill explained.

"Well, the hell with all of you. Good-bye!" she said, and stormed away.

A month or so later, Merrill and his colleagues attended the meeting where Stahlman gave her landmark talk. She used brand new slides. They were clear, with data precisely presented, and crucial points highlighted.

"She never mentioned it to me and I never mentioned it to her," Merrill said, "but we've been best friends ever since."[14]

Stahlman's esteem in the scientific community skyrocketed with the birth of neonatology in the 1960s. At Vanderbilt, she ruled the neonatal intensive care unit (NICU) with an iron glove; she was the supreme commander over the treatment and management of any premature babies who were brought into her hospital. As such, she presented both a blessing and a curse to her chairman, Amos Christie. Although intensely loyal to each other, Christie and Stahlman had no shortage of skirmishes. For one thing, Christie resisted the whole philosophy of pediatric subspecialties and Stahlman was an unapologetic subspecialist.

Christie's daughter Linda Moynihan, who has remained friends with Stahlman through the years, said, "She'd scream at Daddy and make him mad. She was very emotional, which you don't get when you first meet Millie. But my mother was very emotional, too, and I think he thought, 'Oh my God, I've got one at work and one at home, too. I can't stand it!'"

As proud as Christie was of Stahlman's research, he was dismayed by how much it cost the department. Bill DeLoache remembered returning to Vanderbilt and seeking Christie's advice after he had set up his pediatric practice group. Christie took him to see the NICU and bragged about Stahlman's achievements.

"I've got a wild bull by the tail," Christie confessed to DeLoache. "She's getting all this notoriety for what she's doing, but she's using up all my department funds. We can't afford it."[15]

Several years later, Stahlman allayed Christie's financial concerns by arranging a fee schedule so that all the babies who came into Vanderbilt with hyaline membrane disease and were studied in the NICU would have their hospital bills paid for by the National Institutes of Health. "The hospital [administration] was happy with that," Stahlman said.[16]

By the mid-1960s, Stahlman's NICU was a fiefdom unto itself. She trained nurses to specialize in the care of neonates, tested new

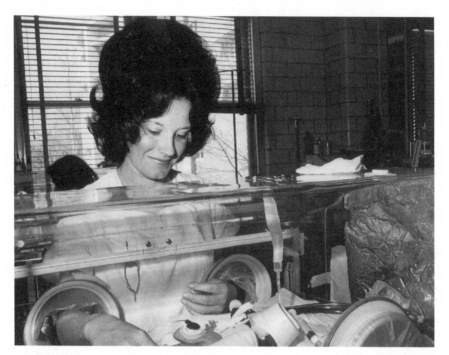

State-of-the-art treatment at Vanderbilt's Neonatal Intensive Care Unit enabled more and more premature infants to survive as healthy children.

respiratory equipment, and conducted increasingly provocative clinical research. With escalating patient loads of smaller and sicker newborns, Stahlman was in need of a vice-admiral for the unit.

She handpicked Dr. Robert Cotton, whom she had trained during his pediatric internship in 1965–66. The Vietnam War was in full throttle then. During his residency, Cotton had opted to follow the Berry Plan, which allowed him to defer his military service until after he'd completed his medical specialty training at the University of Virginia in Charlottesville. When he finished, he planned to enter the air force. Stahlman intervened. She'd arrived in Charlottesville to attend a conference and ran into Cotton at a cocktail party. She asked him what his plans were after he finished his residency. When he told her he would be going into the air force to serve his two-year military commitment, Stahlman sprang into action. Those plans would not do.

Stahlman tracked down another colleague of hers at the party who was in the army and worked at the Walter Reed Army Institute of Research. "Can't you do something for this guy?" she demanded. "He shouldn't just go into the air force and treat snotty noses!"

"Whereupon," said Cotton, "having been ordered, they arranged to get me out of the air force and into the army and assigned me to his office at Walter Reed. I kind of had no other choice. It was preordained somehow that I would come back and do a fellowship with her in neonatology."[17]

Cotton finally completed his military obligations in 1972. He returned to Vanderbilt on September 8, a date he remembers vividly. He had hoped to begin on September 1, but it had taken a week for him to go through all the processing to be honorably discharged from the army. By the time he finally had his papers in order, he was thrilled to be heading back to Nashville. After all those years of waiting to return to Vanderbilt, he had assumed his mentor would give him a warm welcome. When Stahlman saw him walk into the unit, however, instead of the expected greeting, she roared, "Where in the HELL have you been?"

From that day forward, Robert Cotton clearly understood the ground rules for the NICU. He has stayed on ever since.[18]

Perhaps without realizing it, Stahlman and her peers were radically changing the nature of medicine. They were using technology to supplement normal physiology and increase the odds of survival. At the same time that machines were changing how medicine was being practiced and understood, consumers were beginning to demand a role in health care decisions. They were viewing medical interventions in terms of patient rights and environmental responsibility and were asserting that they wanted to be informed about procedures.

"So you had the train of medicine in terms of science, technology and power going one way," explained ethicist Dr. Stuart Finder. "You also had the dawn of people starting to say, 'We want to have some control over what happens to us,' especially as the new technology raised new questions." In pediatrics, this social dynamic led to an emerging mentality among medical providers that children are not little adults and should not be treated as such.[19]

Coupled with this new way of thinking was governmental intercession in the form of social programs. In the 1960s, changes were afoot nationally, locally, politically, and socially that would profoundly affect Middle Tennessee, Vanderbilt, and the Junior League Home for Crippled Children. Events in these unsettled and unsettling times would eventually reopen the debate about building a children's hospital. The counterculture of the turbulent 1960s had not overtaken Nashville as it had in other cities. But the rigid grip of Old South traditionalism was beginning to loosen.

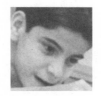

The Medical
Paradigm Shifts | 11

"At the Tennessean *we kept running stories about the three candidates who were in the running to be the new Chancellor of Vanderbilt University. But Alec Heard was impressive and had done his thesis on the politics of the South. Anyway, we had two or three stories saying, 'Alec Heard, the liberal head of the political science department at the University of North Carolina . . .'*

Jimmy [Stahlman] had a lock on anything that was going on at Vanderbilt and we were just picking up the pieces. Finally one of the board members called us and said, 'Please, could you just stop calling Alec Heard a liberal? Every time you do, we have trouble with Jimmy.'"

**—John Seigenthaler, former publisher
of the** Tennessean **newspaper**

hile the members of the Junior League of Nashville were waiting for the new Nashville Children's Hospital to get off the ground (unaware that it never would), they began making plans for utilizing the Crippled Children's Home on White Avenue, still assuming they would turn their patients over to the care of the state. Attuned to the timbre of the times, members had already begun taking an interest in the well-being of children with emotional disturbances. They intended to reach children suffering from abuse and neglect and had opened the Mental Health Center on the property, later known as the Dede Wallace Center (now Centerstone). Beginning in 1957, the Junior League had contributed fifteen thousand dollars a year to the operation of the Dede Wallace Center, as well as continuing to run the Home.

In the early 1960s, with plans in the works for a regional children's hospital, the commissioner of the State Department of Mental Health approached the Junior League about converting the Home on White Avenue, located next to the Dede Wallace Center, into a residential treatment facility for emotionally disturbed youngsters. As plans for the community hospital looked more and more uncertain, the membership grew nervous about jumping too soon. They were unwilling, as Ethel Walker said, "to thrust the children into the snow." Consequently, the Junior League terminated their negotiations with the state and voted to continue their convalescent care program as they had in the past.

"Although we would like to have done everything for the emotionally disturbed children, our first commitment is to the children now under our care. And we feel this is in the best interest of everyone concerned," League President Mary Lee Manier explained to the disappointed state commissioner of mental health.[1]

As a fallback, the Junior League Executive Committee petitioned the Joint Commission on the Accreditation of Hospitals to grant them full hospital accreditation, explaining that with the influx of seriously ill patients and the dramatic decrease in their average length of stay (from eighteen months to thirty-eight days), the Home now functioned more as a hospital than as a convalescent unit. If accredited, the Junior League could begin accepting third-party payments. In May 1962, they received national accreditation for a period of three years.[2] League members had reason to celebrate. Three years would certainly buy them plenty of time in which to transfer their children to a more suitable facility. Or so they thought.

In 1962, Mary Lee Manier became a sustaining member of the Junior League and turned over the mantle of the presidency to her successor, Mary Louise Tidwell. Throughout all the tense negotiations and political salvos about building a children's hospital, the League had maintained its revered stature in the surrounding community, and Middle Tennesseans continued to contribute generously to the Crippled Children's Home. The Palm Sunday Paper Sale raked in upwards of $170,000 a year, making it one of the most profitable door-to-door fund-raisers in the nation, thanks to the legwork of League members and the Al Menah Shriners.

Word soon got back to the national Shriner headquarters about the astounding sums Middle Tennesseans were raising for this charitable cause. The national Shriner group decided that, since they also sponsored hospitals for children, they deserved a cut of the revenues. Al Menah Potentate John Walley sent a letter to the Junior League requesting that the League make a financial donation to the Shrine Hospital in Lexington, Kentucky. The Shriners requested a sum of money from the Paper Sale "above that which is required to meet a reasonable and realistic operating budget" for the Home in Nashville. The purpose, the letter said, was to increase "the incentive of the members of the Al Menah Temple to raise a larger amount of money in the Paper Sale than is currently being realized."[3]

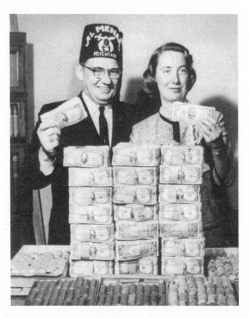

When Mary Louise Tidwell presented the proposal to the Junior League membership, they immediately balked, citing three problems with the proposal. First, the Paper Sale was successful because contributors knew that every penny was going to benefit crippled children housed in a local facility. Second, many Nashvillians were unfamiliar with the Shrine Hospital in Lexington and wouldn't feel compelled

With the Palm Sunday Paper Sale raising around $200,000 a year, the national Shrine organization lobbied to have part of that money go out-of-state to its Shrine Hospitals (left to right: Potentate Raymond Leathers and "Chippy" Pirtle).

to donate to it. Finally, the Junior League of Nashville was not chartered to send funds out of state, nor were they willing to intimate that they were raising more money than they needed by sending a portion of it elsewhere.

The membership adopted a resolution rejecting the proposal, but asking the Al Menah Temple to continue the "magnificent support it has rendered for over thirty years to the crippled children of Middle Tennessee. . . ."

Tidwell continued, "Further, the Board wants conveyed to Al Menah Temple the League's sincere desire to preserve the cordial relationship that has always existed between our two organizations."[4]

The controversy touched off a torrent of bitterness between the two long-standing partners. Yet, when Palm Sunday rolled around again the following year, the Shriners turned out in full force, as they always had, to help raise money for the Junior League Home.

The demise of the proposed children's hospital and the abatement of the lunch counter sit-ins, which had moved en force to other cities, meant that the Vanderbilt board could turn its attention to a pressing matter—the naming of a new Chancellor. Harvie Branscomb had put in seventeen years at the helm of a university that was careening towards distinction, and it was time for someone else to step up and take charge. Trustees initiated a recruitment campaign and began to woo Alexander Heard, dean of the graduate school at the University of North Carolina. Heard had a reputation as a consensus builder and was a proponent of freedom of expression. In other words, he seemed to be someone who could wend his way through the disparate factions at Vanderbilt and still get things accomplished.

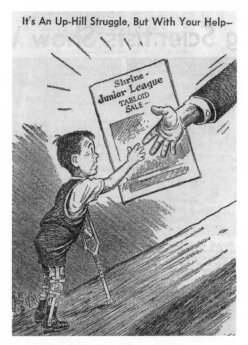

Rival newspapers the Nashville Banner *and the* Nashville Tennessean *could agree on little, except, as shown by this March 1970 cartoon in the* Banner, *support for the Palm Sunday Paper Sale.*

John Seigenthaler was an editor at the *Tennessean* while the search was under way. The *Tennessean* and James Stahlman's *Banner* engaged in a heated scramble to be the first to announce who among the top candidates would take over Branscomb's job. Because of this fierce competition between the dailies, the Board of Trust accidentally tipped its hand.

Seigenthaler recalled:

> At the *Tennessean* we kept running stories about the three candidates who were in the running to be the new Chancellor of Vanderbilt University. But Alec Heard was impressive and had done his thesis on the politics of the South. Anyway, we had two or three stories saying, "Alec Heard, the liberal head of the political science department at the University of North Carolina . . ."
>
> Jimmy [Stahlman] had a lock on anything that was going on at Vanderbilt and we were just picking up the pieces. Finally one of the board members called us and said, "Please, could you just stop calling Alec Heard a liberal? Every time you do, we have trouble with Jimmy."[5]

And thus reporters at the *Tennessean* had a strong clue that Heard was going to be the board's first choice.

One of Heard's greatest assets as Chancellor was that he was a gifted orator. He could mesmerize an audience with his sonorous, well-crafted delivery. "Nobody on the board could argue with Alec, because Alec was so eloquent," said historian Ridley Wills. "Heard was a moderate, and Vanderbilt retained a placid, conservative ambiance throughout the '60s, because he was head of the pack."[6]

Shortly after he became Chancellor, Heard gave a speech to the Junior League about the crucial need for investment in education, particularly in higher education, in Tennessee. "Despite the progress made . . . we can properly conclude . . . that the per capita educational income of Tennessee, at all educational levels, is too low," he told the women. "Our problem is really the problem of our whole Southern region. We need to lift ourselves by our own economic bootstraps, and this is painfully hard to do. . . . The best investment a community can make is in the education of its youth. . . ."[7]

Heard had moved to Nashville precisely when the local leadership was appealing to its citizenry to put an end to the Balkanization that was defining the community. At that time, incorporated satellite cities like Belle Meade, Berry Hill, and Oak Hill functioned as separately governed entities, and more neighborhoods were moving in that direction. Startled by the irrevocable trend towards suburban isolationism in the 1950s, "the politicians, planners, and academicians of Nashville"[8] had attempted, but failed, to steer the city towards a consolidated government. According to Vanderbilt professor Daniel Grant, by 1962, Nashville stood "on the brink of metropolitan disintegration."[9]

Remarkably, even the *Banner* and the *Tennessean* paused in their ongoing squabbles and agreed on this issue. Nashville was ripe for a mass exodus from the city center, which would subsequently be followed by urban decay, unless it implemented a shared tax base drawn from a range of economic classes and used it to shore up the inner city. On June 28, 1962, local leaders once again brought forth the item for a vote, and this time 57 percent of voters approved the referendum.

"Consolidated government was an incredibly important change," historian Ridley Wills said. "That referendum enabled Nashville to jump ahead of its peers. If we had not had Metro government, this city would today be surrounded and strangled by eight or ten incorporated cities, leaving an inner city core of poor and troubled people."[10]

For the people of Nashville, the movement to share tax revenues among all the adjoining locales led

Chancellor Alexander Heard arrived at Vanderbilt in 1963 and quickly gained a reputation as a consensus builder.

to a unification of purpose and a sense of interconnection that had been previously missing. Chancellor Heard quickly became aware that a chain of like-minded Conestoga wagons now encircled Vanderbilt's mid-town campus; it was time that the university set aside the war wounds of the past and learned to get along with its contiguous communities. He appointed Dean Randy Batson to improve relations between the community and the Medical Center. Heard knew that if he could get the locals to respect and to like Vanderbilt, they would begin to support it financially.

"It was hard times," recalled Batson's wife, Bennie.

> The only money that came in was what Randy solicited as a fund-raiser. He was not only the dean, but the fund-raiser. He wore about twelve different caps and did more jobs than one man could possibly handle alone. Randy was gone a lot, always on the road to try to get money. I remember it as being such a hard time.[11]

Amos Christie came up with one solution to help solve community relations. Part of Vanderbilt's problem in patient care during that period was due to an acute nursing shortage in Middle Tennessee. Sick, frightened, and lonely patients wanted to interact with competent, caring nurses, who were in short supply in the immediate area. Christie suggested to his buddy Dr. John Shapiro, chairman of the Department of Pathology, that since Meharry had closed its nursing program a few years earlier, Vanderbilt could begin training young black women to become professional nurses. Christie wrote of his idea:

> There is a large backlog of superior young Negro girls of college caliber who find it difficult to have professional opportunity for economic advancement and self-improvement. If Vanderbilt could offer these young girls opportunities for nurses training it would in my judgment be a step in the right direction. . . . It is such a good idea there must be something wrong with it.[12]

Christie acknowledged that there would be government funding for an initiative with such "national appeal," and that the major drawback would be the likely housing crisis that the plan would precipitate, meaning that both white and black nurses-in-training would have to share dorm space.[13] In the fall of 1964, Vanderbilt's undergraduate campus had just begun to integrate. Christie understood that for its survival, the Medical Center had to continue moving in a direction of racial harmony. Already, the city of Nashville was awkwardly lumbering forward in that same direction.

Similarly, forces of change designed to improve the general welfare were taking place all over the nation, including Washington, D.C. Inspired by the success of Social Security, the United States Congress began to consider establishing programs of government-sponsored health insurance for the elderly, indigent, and "medically indigent," those whose incomes fell above the poverty level but were not high enough to afford costly medical care. In 1965, Congress signed into law two groundbreaking programs—Medicare, providing federally financed health insurance for the elderly, and Medicaid, which provides health care for the poor and is administered by individual state governments through a program of combined state and federal funding.[14]

For charity-laden institutions like Vanderbilt, the Medicare-Medicaid act was an unexpected windfall. It led to a precipitous drop in the number of uninsured patients that university physicians had to treat, which immediately boosted the institution's bottom line. On the other hand, for the newly accredited Junior League Home for Crippled Children, Medicaid reimbursements generated mounds of paperwork, all of which had to be sorted and sifted by part-time volunteers. League members were thrust into a bureaucratic nightmare as they tried to navigate esoteric state and federal channels in order to receive payments for patients at the Home. Once again, they desperately sought a lifeline.

Late in 1966, the indefatigable George Holcomb met Amos Christie in the hallway of Vanderbilt Hospital. "Dr. Christie, have you changed your mind about the children's hospital?" Holcomb asked. "We really need a children's hospital here with first-class services. I know the community will support it."

With a sigh, Christie answered the surgeon, "Why don't you write Randy [Batson]?"[15]

Christie was now sixty-three years old, and he was getting tired. Medicine as he once knew and loved it was disappearing, having slid onto a course he found murky and hard to understand. Baptist and St. Thomas Hospitals were once again considering opening up more beds for children, which would slice into the limited pediatric census at Vanderbilt.[16] As a result of the newly implemented Vanderbilt Professional Practice Plan, academic physicians were operating on a bold new compensation scheme tied to clinical practice—an arrangement that directly conflicted with the sacred tenets set forth by William Osler and Abraham Flexner. Vanderbilt doctors were expecting to be paid salaries still lower but more in line with private practitioners.[17] Christie's motto had always been, "If you're too busy to go fishing, you're too busy." The upcoming generation of what he considered angst-ridden, overtrained specialists and subspecialists was demanding higher incomes and world-class resources. They were clearly too busy to go fishing.

In addition, students were showing up for interviews to medical school dressed like street urchins. Highly qualified women candidates pulled their hair into cutesy pigtails and appeared in his office wearing miniskirts and go-go boots. Men with long hair and sideburns, ranked at the top of their classes, slouched into the conference room to talk about their ambitions.[18] The halo around academic medicine was beginning to evaporate for Amos Christie. In November 1966, Christie told Dean Batson that he was planning to retire in two years when he reached age sixty-five and suggested that the administration begin a search for his replacement in order to ensure a smooth transition.[19]

Meanwhile, Holcomb did as suggested and wrote a letter to Dean Batson. The chief was giving in. He had resisted as long as he could. If Holcomb could get Batson to agree to build a children's hospital, Christie would go along with it. At least he could take some comfort in the knowledge that it would be Vanderbilt's project. Holcomb also believed that Christie would embrace the idea once he got used to it. In his letter, Holcomb updated his earlier data about the shortage of pediatric beds and equipment and laid out, point by point, the reasons why Nashville would be well-served by a freestanding community children's hospital. Ideally, a separate, independent board of directors comprised of representatives from all the major hospitals in town would oversee operation of the facility. Fund-raising sources, such as the Junior League/Shriners' Palm Sunday Paper Sale and the Junior Chamber of Commerce's Clinic Bowl, could be redirected towards the new hospital for children.[20]

If Batson ever felt disinclined to consider Holcomb's proposal, he was forced to take it under advisement due to another phenomenon occurring in town, which was particularly horrific to the old guard at Vanderbilt. Across West End Avenue, respected cardiologist Dr. Thomas Frist Sr. had latched onto a budding trend in American medicine—the concept of a for-profit health care facility. In the early 1960s, Frist spearheaded a group of physician-investors interested in building a nursing home next to Centennial Park. Several years later, he and other shareholders converted the property into what became known as Park View Hospital, the city's first for-profit hospital.

Although economic drivers had always been a component of medicine, Frist and his colleagues were unabashedly using them as a source of motivation. While Vanderbilt and Meharry sought out practicing physicians and researchers on the one hand and financial donors on the other, Park View was working hard to solicit individuals willing to simultaneously serve as investors, share-holders, and practitioners.

In the early days of Park View Hospital, which was underutilized because patients and referring physicians had not entirely bought into the idea, the Junior League Executive Committee approached its administrators about renting a couple of floors in the hospital for the treatment of crippled children and moving the Junior League Home there. After serious contemplation, Park View owners decided to allow the Home to transfer its patients there, under the condition that the contract would be restricted to two years, which would allow Park View time to build up its adult census.

Junior League member Joanne Bailey said, "We flirted with that idea for a while. The problem was that we didn't know what was going to happen after that. They didn't want us forever." Afraid they'd eventually "be left high and dry" and scurrying to find another place to house the children, League members turned down the offer.[21]

By 1967, Frist was ready to turn Park View Hospital over to the Metropolitan Government of Davidson County. When that deal fell through, he consulted Jack Massey, who had earlier been the fund chairman for the defunct children's hospital. Frist's son, Tommy Frist Jr., had just returned to Nashville after completing his two-year military obligation as a flight surgeon. Rather than reentering his residency program at Vanderbilt, Tommy Frist convinced his father and Jack Massey that they ought to form a partnership and establish a hospital company. Frist Jr. had become impressed by the rise of American franchises—such as Holiday Inn, the brainchild of Kemmons Wilson, the father of one his Vanderbilt fraternity brothers, and Kentucky Fried Chicken, where Massey had made a fortune as an early investor. Frist Jr. suggested that the three of them could do for hospitals what KFC had done for chicken. In 1968, the triumvirate founded Hospital Corporation of America (HCA), with Park View Hospital the company's first acquisition.[22]

The Vanderbilt medical faculty considered it one thing for doctors to invest in a struggling hospital. It was quite another for them to use patients as cogs in a business franchise. They knew that executives often made quick, even ruthless business decisions to close down money-losing, poorly performing facilities in a franchise chain. Would they also be willing to coldheartedly shut down hospitals they'd purchased? Many began to view HCA physicians, who'd been their neighbors and friends, as opportunists and traitors to the profession.

Tommy Frist later told *Vanderbilt Magazine*:

> I went to my attending, [surgery chairman] Dr. Scott at Vanderbilt, and I still have nightmares when I think about telling that gray-haired old man that I wasn't coming back to my residency program because I was going to start a for-profit hospital company. He made me feel like a heathen.[23]

During the interim when Randy Batson was in search of a new person to chair the Department of Pediatrics, which was taking longer than he'd hoped, the paradigm of medicine had shifted and transmogrified around him. HCA altered not only the playing field, but also the rules of the game. Years later, Jack Massey would gloat, "Vanderbilt spent many dollars to try to get us out of business."[24]

It was in this milieu that David Karzon, a modest, soft-spoken pediatrician and scientist from Buffalo, New York, came to look at the Vanderbilt job. He scrutinized the Medical Center that had been renovated and added on to in fits and starts so that the building was now a haphazard configuration of mazelike corridors. He spent three hours with Chancellor Heard, ambling among the magnolias, redbuds, and dogwoods that lined the undergraduate campus, discussing philosophy and science. He also spoke to the team of Vanderbilt physicians, who still exuded an idealism about their goals as investigators and the value to the world of medical research.

His talk with Chancellor Heard made a tremendous impression, convincing him that Vanderbilt was a university ready for new ideas and eager for an infusion of innovative thinkers. On the way to the airport, Karzon sat in the backseat of a chauffeur-driven car listening to Dean Batson give his sales pitch and trumpet all the reasons why he should come to Nashville.

"May I build a children's hospital?" David Karzon asked him.

Randy Batson took a deep breath. "Yes," he answered.

That night Karzon returned to his home in New York and spoke excitedly with his wife, Allaire. "I accepted the job at Vanderbilt," he told her. "We're going to move to the South."[25]

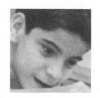

A New Chief, New Plans | 12

"[David Karzon] told me he came here because Vanderbilt was a good medical school that desperately wanted to be great. There was no money. That wasn't the incentive. He was proud of what Vanderbilt was doing on such a small budget and proud of himself for knowing an opportunity when he saw one."

—Dr. William Altemeier, recalling his conversation with Dr. David Karzon, shortly after Karzon joined the Vanderbilt faculty

If the oddsmakers had been laying down bets in the fall of 1968, they would have given 10 to 1 that David Karzon didn't stand a chance. He was everything that Amos Christie was not—quiet, humble, meticulous, intensely private, and, by his own admission, achingly naïve. He was also an outsider—in fact, a Yankee. Yet, all of these traits would ultimately serve Karzon well when he became chairman of pediatrics at Vanderbilt. In order for the Medical Center to bridge the divide it had with the Nashville community, it would need to be represented by someone prone more to listening than talking. Karzon was a listener.

The youngest of four siblings, he grew up in New York City where his father owned a garment factory that made alpaca coats. Young David was an unusual city kid in that he often traveled alone on the subway, taking it to the farthest stop north of the city where he'd debark and walk to Westchester; there he'd spend his afternoons collecting toads, lizards, frogs, or fish. Carefully, he'd smuggle his prized finds back to his family's small apartment and try to keep them alive in the bathtub. His mother was tolerant of his hobbies, his sisters less so. When the Depression hit, Karzon's father lost his factory, throwing the family into sudden intractable poverty. Luckily for David, however, they moved to Bridgeport, Connecticut, which was much closer to the water so he could continue collecting and studying creatures of the natural world.

While a senior at Stuyvesant High School, a rigorous school for math and science students, the future doctor was accepted at Yale University. That same year his father died, leaving the family in worse financial shape than ever. Although his siblings had already made it to college, Karzon's mother could not possibly afford the tuition at Yale. Determinedly, she took the one asset left to her by her husband, an insurance policy, and cashed it in, which provided her youngest son with enough money for his first year of college. It was the best she could do.

As expected, the money ran out after that first year, so Karzon decided to transfer to Ohio State University and study wildlife conservation. He enjoyed the field so much that he continued on and received a master's degree in the subject, writing his thesis on the cottontail rabbits of Ohio. Fortunately, the hunters at that time were interested in those rabbit populations as well, so his research was well-funded. He traveled across the state of Ohio, living with farmers, sometimes sleeping in barns, examining the habits of cottontail rabbits.

Although he'd enjoyed his master's project, Karzon soon realized that he had selected a finite topic. If he really wanted to pursue grant-supported research, he would need to begin studying humans, which meant he would have to go to medical school. He ran into one problem—he had never taken many of the prerequisite medical school courses, such as Latin, German, or the customary advanced sciences. Despite these insufficiencies, he presented an intriguing application and was asked to come for an interview at Johns Hopkins Medical School. He persuaded the assistant dean that he could handle the medical school curriculum and was accepted at Johns Hopkins on the condition that he not only complete the required classes, but that he also receive tutoring in the courses in which he was deficient.

"It is clear you do not know Latin," his Latin professor huffed at the end of Karzon's first year of medical school. "You pass."

Midway through his first year of medical school, Karzon once again found himself so broke that he knew he would have to drop out until he could save enough money to return. Fate intervened. On December 7, 1941, the Japanese attacked Pearl Harbor. The United States declared war and the army realized it was going to need doctors. Karzon was drafted into the army and became a private first-class, and the United States government paid for him to continue his medical school training in exchange for two years of military service.

During his internship year at Johns Hopkins, he studied under famed physician Dr. Warfield Longcope. At that time, many of the faculty had left to join the war effort. The elderly Longcope, who headed up the Osler Medical Clinic, was vastly understaffed and his house officers were pushed to the limit of endurance. Working day and night at the hospital, Karzon became ill. Longcope suggested he take a week off for Christmas, go to Florida, and try to rebuild his strength. In December of 1945, Karzon headed to Sarasota.

Relaxing on the beach, Karzon noticed a teenage boy wearing a Yale T-shirt struggling to carry several sacks of lunch to his family, so he offered to help. While being introduced to the Urban family, Karzon couldn't help but notice the boy's sister, a pretty brown-haired girl who was enrolled in Yale Law School. Allaire Urban was too busy studying for exams to pay much attention to the shy, scrawny intern talking to her family on the beach, but that night Karzon joined the Urban family for dinner and sparks flew between David and Allaire—the kind of chemistry that can't be reproduced in the lab. At the end of that vacation, he returned to Johns Hopkins and she to Yale.

Over the next five months, the two saw each other only inter-mittently when one or the other could get away for a long weekend. Then in May of 1946, Karzon took the train up to New Haven, Connecticut, and told his girlfriend that the army had called him up and he was going to be sent overseas. They decided to marry right away. The wedding was held within twenty-four hours, in the middle of the day at the home of the Urban's family lawyer, and performed by the town mayor. In order to complete the paperwork, Allaire's father paid off the town clerk by giving him a case of whiskey in exchange for predating their marital application. After a three-day honeymoon, the new Mrs. Karzon went back to law school and her husband to Baltimore, where he was told that plans had changed. The army needed him to stay stateside.

"I was ready to throttle him because I'd always wanted to have a white wedding," Allaire Karzon said. "He never went overseas and I never had a white wedding. But I did go back and complete law school."[1]

Karzon, in turn, was sent to Aberdeen Proving Grounds in Maryland to fulfill his military requirements, seeing his wife only on intermittent weekends when she could commute by train. After his army tour was complete, the couple was finally able to live together in the same city. He accepted the position of chief resident at Baltimore's Sydenham Hospital, a medical center that specialized in communicable diseases such as polio, measles, scarlet fever, small pox, chicken pox, and diphtheria,[2] which were raging across the country in the 1940s. In fact, diphtheria was so pandemic that Karzon never left the grounds of the hospital in the first six months that he worked there. He and his wife lived in a house next to the hospital. Since surgeons were in short supply and since the war demanded flexibility, Karzon, whose specialty was internal medicine, took call every other night and performed all the tracheotomies for the children with diphtheria.

Karzon's experience at Sydenham triggered an interest in two areas that he would pursue for the rest of his medical career—research in infectious diseases and the compassionate treatment of children. To fulfill the first passion, he journeyed across town and returned to Johns Hopkins to begin a medical research fellowship in the study of Newcastle disease, a contagious viral infection affecting all species of birds, including poultry.

In the meantime, Allaire Karzon was having trouble finding a job. She had graduated in the top 10 percent of her Yale Law School class, but Baltimore in the late 1940s was not yet willing to hire a female attorney. She recalled, "[Attorneys in the Baltimore law firms] told me, 'Ladies don't practice law!'"

Her options limited, she spent the next year commuting to Washington to work for the Department of Justice, which willingly hired women. In 1950, she was pregnant with their first son, David "Deke" Karzon Jr., so she quit her job and stayed home to help her husband with his research. At that time, Karzon was conducting experiments on chickens in order to formulate a vaccine for Newcastle disease. This required going into the lab at certain times of the day or night and exsanguinating them (draining their blood).

Together they would make nighttime runs into the laboratory, where Karzon would instruct his wife to hold the chicken while he slit its throat and captured its blood. "Don't worry," he told her, confidently, "there's nothing to it."

"I had to hold these dying chickens as he exsanguinated them. And they screeched and writhed in my hands as the life was pouring out of them," Allaire Karzon recalled. "I did that just a few times and then I decided I didn't want anything to do with medicine anymore."

Throughout his fellowship, Karzon couldn't shake the memory of those sick children he'd cared for at Sydenham, young bodies ravaged by terrible infectious diseases. So he decided to pursue an additional residency in pediatrics at Cornell Hospital in New York City.

When they moved to New York, Allaire Karzon finally landed in a location receptive to the concept of a practicing female attorney. She accepted a job in the legal department of RCA and thrived there; whereupon her husband completed his pediatric training and chose to relocate one more time, assuming his first faculty position at Buffalo Children's Hospital in upstate New York. Once again, his wife was out pounding the pavement searching for a firm willing to hire a young female lawyer. Eventually, a large local practice group offered her a job.

"When I went to Buffalo in 1952, they were very reluctant to hire a woman," Allaire Karzon recalled. "It helped that I was married and had a child, which seemed to them stable and safe. I was the sole woman for a long time, and rose to junior, and then senior partner in the firm."[3]

While Allaire Karzon was blazing trails in the legal world, the family welcomed their second child, daughter Elizabeth. Meanwhile, David Karzon was immersing himself in the field of pediatric infectious diseases. He began studying the poliomyelitis virus and collaborated with esteemed Harvard Medical School researcher Dr. John Enders. Enders, along with his colleagues Dr. Frederick Robbins and Dr. Thomas Weller, won the 1954 Nobel Prize in medicine for their seminal discovery of a technique for growing the polio virus in the laboratory. Their research laid the groundwork for scientists Jonas Salk and Albert Sabin to develop vaccines against polio that would ultimately eradicate the disease from the Western world.

A year later, while Amos Christie, Randy Batson, and Pete Riley were celebrating the announcement of the efficacy of the polio vaccine at the Noel Hotel in Nashville, David and Allaire Karzon were headed to Geneva, Switzerland, to attend a celebration hosted by Basil O'Connor, president of the National Foundation for Infantile Paralysis, in honor of all the scientists whose investigations contributed to the landmark discovery.

With polio on the wane, Karzon turned his attention to vaccines for influenza, mumps, and chicken pox, in addition to maintaining his teaching and clinical responsibilities at Buffalo Children's Hospital. His success in the laboratory began to attract the attention of academicians around the country. By 1967, having worked in Buffalo for sixteen years, David Karzon was considered to be a hot commodity in the world of physician-scientists. He could have had his pick of a faculty role at any number of fine medical institutions, which is why some people were stunned when he announced that he was leaving Buffalo to head up the pediatric department at Vanderbilt University Hospital. His colleagues knew he was ready for a challenge, but that small institution in the belly of the South seemed less like a challenge than a swan dive into dark, shallow water. David Karzon did not possess the personality of a risk-taker and to those in the Northeast, and even to a number of folks in the South, accepting a position at Vanderbilt seemed like an unnecessarily risky career move.

Karzon could not have articulated to his colleagues the deep-seated feelings behind his leap of faith. In all truth, he took the job because he was a visionary. His work on submicroscopic proteins inspired him to dream big. He had a vision that aspects of medicine were simply waiting to be explored, and that there were better ways for children to receive medical care and for residents to be trained. He wanted parents to be included in the decision-making process regarding medical options available to their children. Karzon chose Vanderbilt because he saw possibilities there. Vanderbilt, among all the universities recruiting him, offered a potter's wheel where he could spin and formulate his ideas.

Even during his residency, Vanderbilt held a strange allure, his wife said, because he viewed it as a "sister" hospital to Johns Hopkins. Physicians and scientists trained at one institution and then left to practice at the other. The flow between the two schools was steady and mutually enriching. For example, Alfred Blalock, the renowned cardiac surgeon, trained at Vanderbilt and then joined the Hopkins faculty. Elliott V. Newman completed his residency at Johns Hopkins and then departed for a research position at Vanderbilt. When Karzon visited Vanderbilt, he felt it exuded "the same aura as Johns Hopkins," his wife remembered.[4]

Later, when Karzon was recruiting physicians to join him in Nashville, he talked about the choices he'd made a few years before. William Altemeier, who would accept Karzon's offer to head the Vanderbilt program in pediatrics at Nashville General Hospital, said, "He told me he came here because Vanderbilt was a good medical school that desperately wanted to be great. There was no money. That wasn't the incentive. He was proud of what Vanderbilt was doing on such a small budget and proud of himself for knowing an opportunity when he saw one."[5]

Karzon accepted the job at Vanderbilt first and then broke the news to his family. To put it mildly, Allaire Karzon was astonished. "I had never been to the South," she said. "I'd never wanted to live in the South. This was very hard on me. At that point I was the only female senior partner in a major law firm in Buffalo. And I had to leave."

David and Allaire Karzon were a power couple before there was such a term. They were also unwavering in their devotion to one another and their support of each other's careers. Allaire flew down to Nashville and informed a local real estate agent that she needed to buy a house that weekend because she had to get back to work on Monday. She looked at several houses and purchased the one that they've lived in for over thirty years.

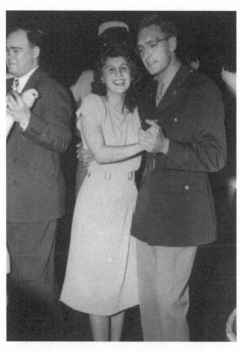

Finding a house in town was easy. Finding Allaire a job in Nashville was substantially trickier. In the late 1960s, very few women practiced law in Tennessee—in fact, many Southerners scoffed at such a notion. Dean Batson knew that David and his wife would come only as a total package, so he called up prominent attorney Henry Hooker, a Vanderbilt supporter and brother to John Jay Hooker, a Democratic politico. The Hooker brothers offered Allaire a job as legal counsel and vice president of their new fran-

During the 1940s, the Karzons were an unusual power couple. David Karzon was a physician, studying infectious diseases in children, and Allaire Karzon was a practicing attorney.

chise, Minnie Pearl's Chicken System—Nashville entrepreneurs' answer to Kentucky Fried Chicken's hugely popular chain of restaurants.

On paper, this position would seem like the perfect open-arms introduction for an out-of-towner to the movers and shakers of Nashville. The founders belonged to a respected family complete with their own gubernatorial candidate in John Jay Hooker. The franchise president, Ed Nelson, had been a leading executive of Commerce Union Bank. Investors ranged from the *Tennessean's* John Seigenthaler and Amon Evans to *Banner* publisher Jimmy Stahlman. Highly regarded attorneys, politicians, and federal judges owned stock in the company, as did its namesake country music star Sarah Cannon (who performed under the stage name Minnie Pearl). When Allaire Karzon joined Minnie Pearl's Chicken System in 1968, it was a darling of Wall Street with hundreds of franchises sold in many locations.[6]

The bubble exploded for Minnie Pearl's Fried Chicken during the same time that David Karzon was attempting to build a children's hospital. The Securities and Exchange Commission began an investigation into alleged fraudulent business practices and Allaire Karzon was called upon to retain a New York law firm to represent the corporation before the SEC. She also had to orchestrate the legal issues involved in compensating franchisees, who were having to close down their restaurants. That period of her life was so hectic, she said, and she felt such tremendous pressure to "prove herself" to the people of Nashville that she rarely had an opportunity to talk to David about the troubles he might be going through with the children's hospital.

She traveled to Washington with Sarah Cannon to testify before a Senate committee that was looking into famous personalities lending their names to dubious franchise operations. Cannon testified that she had not sold her name and had been personally involved in the business and, in fact, had her own office in the headquarters building. Senators were uncomfortable facing down two demure, seemingly innocent ladies.

"They gave us a very easy time," Allaire said. "If she'd had some big powerful male attorney, they might have been tougher."

When Minnie Pearl's Chicken System folded in 1970, Allaire formed a partnership with attorney James F. Neal (renowned for having prosecuted mob boss Jimmy Hoffa) and Aubrey Harwell. Together they opened up the downtown office of Neal, Karzon, and Harwell.

With Allaire thus preoccupied, David Karzon was also becoming acclimatized to the idiosyncrasies of the Nashville and Vanderbilt communities. Although Amos Christie had recently retired, after twenty-five years as chairman, he was still essentially running the show. Amos and Margaret Christie welcomed the new chairman and his wife to town and generously introduced them to friends, but Allaire was busy and David was, by nature, introverted.

Explains Robert Merrill in his biography of Amos Christie:

> . . . Dr. Karzon became aware of the revered status that AC [Christie] had attained within the medical school and parts of the community so that he was inclined to be very careful how he expressed any difference of opinion. By contrast, AC was not content to remain silent as Dr. Karzon proceeded along lines that AC thought were ill-advised . . . Fortunately, there was never any unpleasant confrontation, but they never went fishing together, either.[7]

Before David Karzon accepted the chairmanship, Dean Batson faced a gnawing dilemma. The main hospital and clinical facilities, built in 1925, were woefully outdated by the 1960s. This limited the number

By the late 1960s, Vanderbilt's medical facilities were outdated, limiting the number of patients who could be admitted, the number of new faculty who could be hired, and the type and quality of research that could be performed.

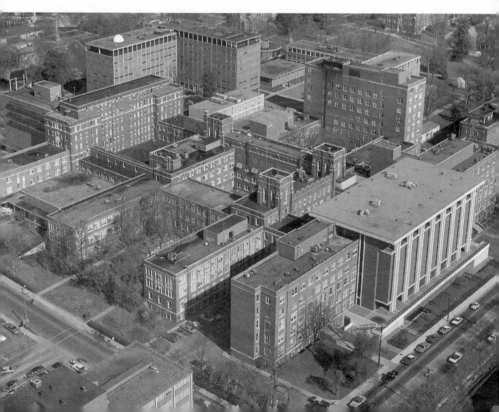

of patients who could be admitted, the number of new faculty who could be hired, and the type and quality of research that could be performed. In his search to fill the slot of pediatric chairman, it became increasingly obvious that every candidate worth consideration was asking for improved space and more resources. The Round Wing was constructed to house pediatrics, but it only served as an addition to the hospital and not a replacement for it. Also, the Vietnam War was pulling young physicians on the faculty away from their hospital duties.

"The situation is that the Selective Service System has grown somewhat rusty and was very poorly prepared for the additional special call for physicians in September of 1965," wrote Dr. Robert C. Berson, executive director of the Association of American Medical Colleges, in response to a complaint by Batson. "As you might imagine, the established system is quite difficult to change."[8]

Soon it appeared that a solution was at hand. The United States Congress, responding to national workforce studies indicating an impending shortage of physicians, passed a bill called the Health Facilities Development Act, to help medical schools develop teaching facilities and to promote an upswing in the number of students applying to medical schools. When Karzon came for his interview and asked if he could build a children's hospital, Batson had said yes because he thought he'd be able to earmark some of those designated funds for a children's hospital. If Vanderbilt could begin planning for construction, he was counting on the community to pitch in and help support it. Batson and his administrative team called in architects, and early stage proposals were piling up in his in-box. Shortly thereafter, however, Congress determined it had met its goals and an increase in doctors was no longer an issue, so it discontinued the Health Facilities Development Act.

"Vanderbilt was left having begun planning for the hospital, but with no money in their pockets to develop it," said James O'Neill.[9]

Congress yanking those funds was like a blow to the stomach for Batson. Randy Batson was a man of his word. Born and raised in the Southern town of Hattiesburg, Mississippi, he was handsome and amiable and he held inherent convictions about honor and honesty. Yet here was David Karzon, who had turned down other offers, on his way to Nashville, moving his family, and expecting to establish a free-standing children's hospital. Batson agonized over having to tell his new chief of pediatrics that Vanderbilt wouldn't have the money to make that possible, after all.

What Dean Batson couldn't appreciate was that word about Vanderbilt's movement towards a children's hospital had already leaked out and was forming cascades of promises and expectations all over town. A groundswell of enthusiasm arose among local surgeons and orthopedists, and they were beginning to recruit physicians to town with the promise of the impending new children's hospital. The new regime at the Junior League began to feel cautiously optimistic, as well.[10] Even Amos Christie, who had allegedly retired, was getting in on the act. He drafted a letter to Batson calling not for a hospital, but rather for "an attractive place [for] quality diagnostic and treatment facilities," and "space for ambulatory care."[11] Batson was being ambushed, unable to hold back the onslaught of interest, knowing he didn't have the funding streams to meet the demands placed upon him.

When Karzon arrived at Vanderbilt in the fall of 1968, Dean Batson regretfully explained to him that although they weren't giving up, financial reasons had forced them to postpone their plans to build a children's hospital anytime in the near future.

Karzon didn't say much in response. He mostly just listened.

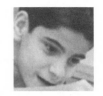

Courting the Community | 13

*"I knew we needed three things to happen
if this was going to work. We'd need the support
of the Junior League, we'd need the support of the
community, and we'd need the support of Vanderbilt.
I way underestimated how easy it would be to get
the support of the community. And I way underestimated
how hard it would be to get the support of Vanderbilt."*

**—Nelson Andrews, first Board chairman of the Children's
Regional Medical Center at Vanderbilt**

In basic science, if all the procedures are carried out according to protocol, there is no such thing as a failed experiment. Sometimes the results are unexpected, often they are disappointing, but they are legitimate results all the same. They provide ammunition for an investigator who then must step back and reconnoiter, rethink the approach to the question, formulate new tactics, and begin anew, sometimes from ground zero.

Fortunately for Vanderbilt, David Karzon thought like a basic scientist. When Randy Batson informed him about the unanticipated funding deficit, Karzon asked him to explain how that had evolved. Batson let him know about earlier discussions in which he and his associate deans had been stymied about what to do. "Why don't we just call what we have [i.e., the pediatric ward] a children's hospital?" Batson had asked.[1]

In fact, Nashvillians had been bandying about the term "children's hospital-within-a-hospital" for nearly a decade, but nobody had figured out how to make it work in practical terms.

There remains some controversy about exactly when the first children's hospital-within-a-hospital actually came to fruition. What is clear, however, is that the concept did work successfully at one time back in the late 1880s, and serendipitously, it occurred at Karzon's old stomping grounds, Buffalo Children's Hospital.

That city's denizens established Buffalo General Hospital in 1858, but the facility offered hospital services to male patients only. Incensed that the city provided no similar facility for females, a group of wealthy philanthropic women formed the Ladies Hospital Association (LHA) and organized a women's ward within the general hospital. Because the women's ward, financed largely by the LHA, was a huge success, the organization later petitioned the hospital board of trust to create a similar ward for the care of children. After the board rejected the proposal, the mayor of the town paid the start-up costs for a children's ward out of his own pocket. In 1884, Buffalo's Children's Ward was born, consisting of two rooms of ten beds each, located in the least desirable space of the building—over the clanging, steamy boiler room.[2]

The people of Buffalo responded generously to the new ward. Wrote one newspaper:

> When the work was well begun gifts poured in so profusely that only a part of the money had to be used for the purpose intended. So many people wished to help furnish a ward for sick and crippled children that their efforts had to be guided to other channels—there was not room enough for all the beds that were proposed to be endowed.[3]

Although the hospital-within-the-hospital filled a need, the arrangement was less than perfect. Board members were vexed that the unit siphoned off charitable dollars from the general hospital. The volunteers of the LHA, who were responsible for running the ward, felt unappreciated and ignored by the trustees, staff, and hospital administration. The LHA came to realize that their novel concept was only a temporary solution. In 1892, they asked the board to move the children's ward to a separate building, but the trustees soundly rejected that idea.

Refusing to be cowed, a committee of women then purchased a red-brick home in Buffalo, renovated it into a small hospital for children, called it Children's Hospital, and admitted nine young patients. Six years later, with the Children's Hospital gaining steam,

Buffalo General finally agreed to move its pediatric patients to a better location within the main building. In 1902, administrators surrendered to pressure by the few remaining women of the LHA still volunteering at the original hospital and gave the organization permission to elect three of its members to serve on the Buffalo General Hospital Board of Trust. In the end, however, the stand-alone facility maintained its brand as "the children's hospital" and won the support of the community, later evolving into modern-day Buffalo Children's Hospital.[4]

When David Karzon learned that he would not be able to build a freestanding children's hospital in Nashville, he decided to try to embed a children's hospital within the university Medical Center, much as the women of the LHA had done. He began a detailed evaluation of the situation at Vanderbilt. The pediatric unit housed a remarkably small number of inpatients. Only four-teen physicians—including Amos Christie, who'd retired, and Randy Batson, who was inundated with admin-istrative duties—were on the department's faculty, with six residents and six interns handling all the caseloads.[5] Some of the pediatricians had stellar clinical skills and reputa-tions as researchers, but because the faculty was so limited, glaring gaps in services plagued the department. Karzon was going to have to beef up the faculty, particularly in the subspecialties.

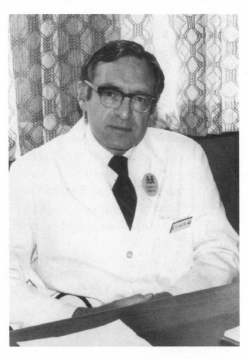

Dr. David Karzon had a new vision for taking care of pediatric patients in Middle Tennessee, which included building a community children's hospital.

Also, the patient load was inadequate for either heavy-duty clinical research or for teaching. One way to increase the census was to

abandon the old rules set up by Christie and give all interested pediatricians in town admitting privileges to Vanderbilt. Another was to join
forces with the surgical team so that pediatric patients could be placed
into a special intensive care unit, much as Mildred Stahlman's premature babies were cared for in the NICU. If more pediatric surgeries
were performed, then more admissions to the unit would follow.

Finally, Karzon understood that he would have to get the
community behind him as he pressed for creating a true children's
hospital within the walls of the existing medical center. That would
entail altering the gestalt of Vanderbilt pediatrics, which wasn't
going to win him any popularity contests. On the other hand,
Karzon reasoned, his primary goal was to provide the best care for
children. Surely, given time, his colleagues would come to appreciate his rationale.

One of Karzon's first questions to Randy Batson was, "Who do I
need to see to get the community's support?"

Batson answered, "Nelson Andrews," and offered to make the call.

Nelson Andrews, who was one of the younger members of the
Vanderbilt Medical Center Board and active in the Chamber of
Commerce, never shied from taking a stance on the tough issues. A
teetotaler, he led the 1967 fight to get liquor by the drink passed in
Nashville, knowing it would attract higher class hotels and restaurants
to the city and raise Nashville's status as a tourist destination.[6] When
Batson phoned him up, he appealed to Andrews's sense of duty to
improve the community.

"Would you talk to David Karzon?" Batson asked. "He's got this
wild idea and I don't know if it has any merit or not, but I do know
that it would get us involved in the community, and we haven't done
too good a job of that so far."[7]

Andrews arranged to meet with the newcomer, and Karzon told
him all about his vision of creating a children's hospital within
Vanderbilt. Andrews had met many department chairs, but he was
not prepared for David Karzon. In those days, said Andrews, "If you
were a department head, you were a god. You were absolutely in
charge. Randy Batson used to say, 'I'm trying to be a tiger tamer. My
biggest job is handling the whip and chair.'"

Karzon, however, was unique. Andrews was surprised by the
chairman's scientific bent, his methodical parsing of the issues, his
lack of egotism. He seemed like "a nerdish pediatric professor,"
Andrews recalled.

"He was very shy," Andrews continued. "David had no ax to grind. He really was not somebody who was trying to get power for power's sake. He probably understood power less than anybody I know. He was the most idealistically motivated person I've ever come upon."

It was just this lack of presumption and self-promotion that convinced Andrews to help. After he received Batson's assurances that he would stand up to the Vanderbilt forces, Andrews proceeded to help Karzon ply the local waters. "I knew we needed three things to happen if this was going to work," Andrews said. "We'd need the support of the Junior League, we'd need the support of the community, and we'd need the support of Vanderbilt. I way underestimated how easy it would be to get the support of the community. And I way underestimated how hard it would be to get the support of Vanderbilt."[8]

David Karzon had already encountered the Junior League when he'd gone to the Home on White Avenue to attend to a sick child. While there, completely unaware of their acrimonious history, he'd asked one of the volunteers what she thought of Vanderbilt. He got an earful in reply. "Vanderbilt is a terrible place!" the woman had told him. "I would never send my children there! Vanderbilt cannot be trusted!"[9] Andrews was now asking Karzon to court these same women and convince them that Vanderbilt could indeed be trusted. For that to happen, Karzon was going to have to meet with the executive board of the League and separately with influential sustaining members, and he was going to have to speak in front of large groups of women to explain his plans.

Karzon had sputtered, "I can't do that!" He was comfortable speaking before his scientific colleagues on research topics, but he never claimed to be skilled at public appeals to a lay audience.

"You gotta do it, David," Andrews insisted. "You've got a bunch of different constituencies out there to deal with."

The businessman made Karzon a deal. If the doctor would figure out "the mechanical part of creating a hospital-within-a-hospital," Andrews would run interference, negotiating with the Junior League and the Shriners and drawing in Nashville's powerbrokers.

Karzon relented but sometimes almost got physically ill before he'd get up to talk.[10] Andrews would go first, and the pediatric chairman would follow, both of them explaining the reasons why the Junior League should throw its political capital with Vanderbilt and invest in Karzon's plan for a hospital-within-a-hospital. Even though he was a Northerner, Karzon's earnestness, candor, and quiet demeanor won over the League's leaders.

Frances Jackson, who was the League president during these 1969–70 discussions about merging the Home with Vanderbilt, recalled an endearing quality about Karzon's personality. "He was very attractive!" she said with a laugh. "And he was personable. I think he caught on to what he was dealing with in an old, staid, established institution. He was very sympathetic and diplomatic. He tried to move slowly and answer questions. He was just a really charming person and easy to get along with."[11]

Which was not to say that the Junior League was quickly won over. Many of the older members expressed concerns that Vanderbilt was akin to the old sci-fi movie *The Blob*, about an amorphous monster that swallows up everything in its path. They worried that if the Home moved onto a floor at Vanderbilt Hospital, the Junior League of Nashville would be in danger of losing its identity. After all, the Home was the organization's primary claim to fame and valued among Middle Tennesseans from all social echelons.

Also, the League would have to handle the delicate matter of the Trust Fund. Money from the Trust was bequeathed specifically for the benefit of the Crippled Children's Home, and members had to be certain that if Trust money went to Vanderbilt, it would be used only for that purpose and only for those patients. For the next two years, arguments over the merger monopolized every meeting of the Junior League.

"It was never a slam-dunk with the Junior League that they were going to go along with this," Andrews said. "David kept telling them that this is the right thing to do for children. That's a hard thing to battle against."

Then another, even stickier issue arose. For decades, generations of Al Menah Shriners had helped the Junior League with its Palm Sunday Paper Sale, much to the consternation of its national headquarters. The implicit understanding had always been that when the Home for Crippled Children eventually closed, interest from the League's Trust would be donated to the Shrine burn hospitals in nearby states. Suddenly, that was appearing less likely because Vanderbilt was angling to get those funds. The Shriners, understandably, were infuriated and deeply hurt.

Meetings between the League and the Shriners sometimes lasted late into the night, Andrews recalled. Soon, the local newspapers smelled a story and reporters began attending and asking pointed questions. Finally, Andrews pulled one journalist aside and said:

> Don't. You can kill this if you want to, but don't do it. This is something good, so don't build up the conflict between the Junior League and the Shrine and the community and the Medical Center. These people are all trying to do something good.

In the end, the media acquiesced and kept the tone of their reports objective and restrained, refraining from adding flames to the already smoldering deliberations.[12]

The arguments were heating up even without the assistance of the newspapers. One night, not long after he'd arrived in town, Karzon invited every pediatrician, board-qualified or not, to his home. In his living room, which overflowed with curious doctors, he announced that he wanted to invite every one of them to become part of Vanderbilt Hospital and part of the clinical faculty, even those who presently didn't have admitting privileges. The guests were astounded.

"And," Karzon added, "I'd like you to teach if you want to and feel qualified," adding that they would be providing a tremendous service to the residents if they'd help acquaint them with the fundamental aspects of taking care of children in private practice.[13]

Soon after, Nelson Andrews's phone was ringing off the hook. "Is this Karzon guy for real?" the pediatricians wanted to know. Andrews assured him that the pediatrics chief was serious.

A short time later, Karzon set up a system for attending that paired Town and Gown (the two communities that make up a university's locale) in the teaching process.[14] Focused on the welfare of the child more than the morass of politics at the university, Karzon believed that the weaker pediatricians would benefit by having access to the academic center, and children would benefit by having house staff and in-house faculty providing care and consultation in addition to their private doctors.

Pediatrician Dr. David Thombs said:

> He told me, "I don't care how bad the person is who admits, by the time he's ready to send that patient home, he'll be a better doctor. He'll get challenged by the house staff and the academic physicians to learn new techniques and approaches. That will be a positive experience for those doctors and ultimately it will serve the children of Tennessee much better."[15]

Eric Chazen explained:

> In other words, the child would get good care whether the doctor knew what was going on or not. It was a win-win situation for everyone. Town physicians developed increased loyalty to Vanderbilt, and by allowing them to admit patients, it quelled the animosity between the "select few" and the others, who no longer went around bad-mouthing Vanderbilt.[16]

Dr. John Herman was one of many Vanderbilt orthopedic residents who rotated through the Junior League Home for Crippled Children. In fact, ortho-pedists and pediatric surgeons initiated the push for a children's hospital in Nashville and only later were joined by local pediatricians. Photo by Jimmy Ellis, Nashville Tennessean.

The influx of town pediatricians went fairly smoothly, except in the area of neonatology. Once Karzon opened up the department to all pediatricians, some of them felt inclined to enter the domain of Millie Stahlman. The field was still in its infancy and evolving, and the children in the NICU were clinging to life by the smallest of margins. Stahlman didn't want general pediatricians "messing around with her babies" when the neonatology physicians were actually the ones providing care, staying up all night, and taking on the liability of making complex decisions. Stahlman faced down Karzon and insisted, "This has to stop!"[17]

To his credit, said Robert Cotton, Karzon called in all the leading private pediatricians in town and informed them they would not be allowed to treat children in the NICU. Cotton said:

They [private pediatricians] were distraught and made all kinds of threats, but he stood his ground. And that's the way it was. They gave up their control of the sick babies, which they should have done. They didn't have any business trying to manage sick premature infants.[18]

With the town physicians admitting patients to Vanderbilt, the pediatrics department quickly outgrew its space. If there was one issue that could ignite tongue-lashings and vociferous name-calling, it was the debate about space. To some, instead of reforming the pediatrics practice, the new pediatric chairman seemed to be trying to build an empire. The powerful old guard wondered, *who is this new guy—this stranger—anyway? What right does he have to wander into town and start gobbling up space for his patients? We're the ones who've paid our dues, working under suboptimal conditions with minimal resources. Why should Karzon get all the real estate?*

Nelson Andrews tried to intervene. He spoke to the hospital leadership and told them that in order for Karzon's vision to work, people were going to have to adopt a new philosophy. They no longer could be so territorial, bureaucratic, and resistant to change. Andrews's comments infuriated the administrator, who insisted that Vanderbilt was renowned for its interdepartmental collegiality and for its number of cross-departmental research publications—which was true. Collegiality was one thing, Andrews shot back, but turf protection was another.

To prove his point, Andrews decided to conduct a little renegade experiment. He and a friend went over to the Medical Center armed with only two items—a measuring tape and a clipboard. They began walking down the hall and into the offices and laboratories. Apologizing to the startled employees for interrupting, one man would bend down to take a measurement along a wall and then call out the numbers, while the other wrote what he said on the clipboard.

Immediately, everyone was in a panic, running over to ask them what they were doing. "We're measuring," Andrews answered.

"What are you measuring for?" they demanded.

"That's something I'm not at liberty to say," he coyly replied.

"We shut the place down!" he gleefully recalled. Within minutes, the administrator for the hospital came barreling down the hallway, demanding to see their work orders. All the employees on the floor were in near hysteria, speculating about what was being torn down for whom and where they'd be forced to move.

"In any educational bureaucracy, if you monkey with somebody's space, you put your life in peril," Andrews said.[19]

Proving his theory did little to stem the swelling outrage against the requirements for Karzon's hospital-within-a-hospital. People's anger was not without justification. The surgeons needed more operating rooms. The psychiatric unit was so shabby it required a complete overhaul. As John Chapman, who was associate dean of the Medical School said at the time, "Departments do not build hospitals, . . . departments build programs."[20]

Heads of other departments began contacting Nelson Andrews to berate him for diverting so many resources into one department. Andrews tried to explain that a children's hospital would heal some of the rifts between Vanderbilt and the community and thereby raise up all the other departments. But his perspective fell on mostly deaf ears.

Throughout all of this philosophical upheaval, Dean Batson was also getting hammered by department chairmen, worried trustees, and prominent members of the community who remained gun-shy about revisiting old war zones. A number of the city's leaders were still feeling the pain from the previous failed attempts. Still, Batson had said he'd support Karzon's dream, and he would not back down from his promise. Slowly, however, Batson began to crumble under the weight of so much pressure and so many obligations.

For a person holding a position of such high authority, Randy Batson possessed one fatal flaw—he was missing a mean streak. Batson was an outstanding clinician, an inventor who'd patented a groundbreaking device, the Batson Box, that improved the function of ventilators for polio victims. While still a young investigator, he'd agreed to take on a huge job in order to mollify the in-house fighting among the Medical Center's faculty and administrators, and he'd achieved that because he was a decent fellow and a peacemaker. Yet as time progressed, more and more papers and responsibilities landed on his desk. Unlike other hospital officials, he was uncomfortable saying no to his superiors and felt duty-bound to take on whatever project he was given. Soon, his health suffered and he began to stagger, unable to sort through the deluge and determine which crisis to address first.

"Randy was like the guy who every day would go out and pick up his calf and put him over the fence. And pretty soon he had a two-thousand-pound bull he was picking up," recalled one of his associate deans, Dr. Tremaine "Josh" Billings. "For the brilliant mind he had, he came to the realization that he was overwhelmed."[21]

Against all odds, meanwhile, Karzon had gained a toehold in the tough inner circle of Vanderbilt. Surgeons like Bill Scott and George Holcomb and orthopedist William Hillman stood up for his novel concept about a children's hospital, as did certain members of the pediatric staff. Karzon also found a unique ally in Dr. Grant Liddle, who had recently been hired to chair the Department of Medicine. Liddle and Karzon worked out a long-term arrangement for recruiting young faculty in spite of budget restraints. Karzon would lend a year's worth of funding support for the new physician, which would give him time to generate his own grant money. In exchange, the young investigator would spend some portion of his workweek seeing pediatric patients.

Said Allaire Karzon, "Usually medicine and pediatrics aren't that close. But those two [Liddle and Karzon] formed a unique alliance between medicine and pediatrics. They had a reciprocal friendship and they agreed on their values. Both of them were loners."[22]

Although it may have seemed at the time that progress was agonizing and intermittent, in truth, the children's hospital was gaining momentum. The dominoes were being set into place, even if the bricks and mortar were not. For someone who moved with such deliberation and caution, in this particular matter Karzon felt propelled by an intransigent sense of urgency. In fact, he kept in his files a quote by the poet Gabriela Mistral: "Many of the things we need can wait. The child cannot. To him we cannot answer 'Tomorrow' . . . his name is 'Today.'"

Karzon recognized that his supporters wouldn't hang with him forever. If he dared to hesitate, he'd lose the dream. A new decade was dawning. The only acceptable option was for Nashville to ring it in by opening its long-awaited children's hospital.

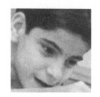

More Than a Place | 14

*"The Children's Hospital is more than geography,
more than a place . . . It consists of all those areas that
care for children in Vanderbilt University Hospital . . .
The Children's Hospital is not bricks and mortar, it is
a way of approaching children's medical needs."*

**—Dr. David Karzon, pediatrician-in-chief
and first medical director of the
Children's Regional Medical Center at Vanderbilt**

In May 1970, David Karzon stood before the Vanderbilt Board of Trust and made a once-in-a-lifetime speech on behalf of the concept of a children's hospital within the university hospital. He stated that just as the child patient population was increasing, the "sound health" of the children of the region was now at stake. Many private hospitals were disbanding their pediatric services, a large percentage of the new for-profit franchised hospitals were not making provisions for children, and the South was falling further behind other regions of the nation in terms of facilities and access to care. Consequently, the primary burden for the delivery of pediatric health care had fallen onto academic medical centers like Vanderbilt.

"To help alleviate the national crisis in child health care facilities and to meet growing regional needs, the Vanderbilt Department of Pediatrics is seeking to establish a Children's Regional Medical Center [CRMC]," he said.[1] Such a center would raise the standard of diagnostic, consultative, and therapeutic services for children. By maximizing the use of available facilities and resources at Vanderbilt University Medical Center, the CRMC could avoid unnecessary and expensive duplication found in a freestanding children's hospital. Also, since a new university hospital was in the planning stages, the CRMC could take over the Round Wing building once the new structure was completed. "In the interim," he concluded, "a Children's Regional Medical Center will be created, in concept and function, in present space."[2]

Boldly, Karzon broached old obstacles, calling for the establishment of a board of directors made up of a combination of medical and nonmedical leaders from Vanderbilt and from the community, with outside members making up the majority of appointees. The Vanderbilt Hospital Medical Board would have final say, granting or denying all final motions by the CRMC Board members.

Although the Vanderbilt Board of Trust was rock-solid conservative, it had recently appointed a few more youthful and forward-thinking members, led by David K. "Pat" Wilson, chairman of Cherokee Insurance Company. Wilson was the youngest trustee around the time that Alec Heard was appointed Chancellor, and he was one of the few board members unfazed by Heard's broadmindedness.

"When Heard first came there was concern on the board because they thought he was too liberal," Wilson said. "And that opinion lasted until most of them died off."

Heard favored Karzon's plans for a children's hospital at Vanderbilt. Pat Wilson, a father of four, worked behind the scenes to get the other trustees to see its potential value to the community and to Vanderbilt. By the time Karzon gave his speech, in fact, the board had already made its decision.[3]

On November 11, 1970, Dean Batson received a letter from the office of Chancellor Heard announcing that the Vanderbilt Board of Trust had approved Karzon's proposal, with the caveat that:

> The Children's Regional Medical Center and activities undertaken through it must be funded in accordance with the standard fiscal policies of the University and no authorization of appropriation therefor [sic] is implied by the adoption of this resolution.[4]

In other words, Karzon was told to proceed if he wanted, but Vanderbilt would not offer any funds towards the creation of a children's hospital. As a chairman, Karzon would still receive designated funds already allocated for the pediatrics department, but anything beyond that he would have to raise himself. To most people, such a lukewarm endorsement by the administration would be a signal to run for the exits. For Karzon and Nelson Andrews, any green light—even a pale one—was a triumph.

Gambling that they were going to receive the go-ahead from the trustees, Andrews had already obtained verbal commitment from many of the local heavy hitters to serve on the CRMC's initial board of directors. Andrews, who agreed to become the first chairman of the board, coaxed a diverse cross section of people to join him in the venture. Among them were local powerbrokers Gilbert Merritt Jr., Lewis Pride, Kirby Primm, John Sloan Jr., Charles Trabue Jr., and James Webb; entrepreneur Jack Massey; Junior League officers Betty Nelson Burch and Mary Stumb; Peggy Steine, an influential member of the local Jewish community; music industry mavens Owen Bradley and Irving Waugh; Hap Motlow from the Jack Daniel Distillery; Amon Carter Evans, who had become publisher of the *Tennessean*;[5]

Community leader Nelson Andrews (left) agreed to serve as the first chairman of the Board of Children's Regional Medical Center. Betty Nelson Burch (right), president of the Junior League, was a key player in the decision to transfer patients at the Crippled Children's Home to Vanderbilt's hospital-within-a-hospital.

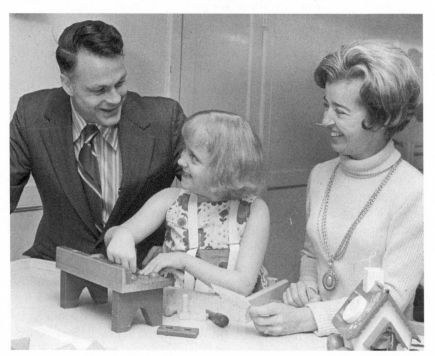

Fred Russell, the nationally renowned sports columnist at the *Banner*; pediatrician James Overall; and, of course, George Holcomb, who was finally within reach of his goal for a community children's hospital.

Comprised of so many respected citizens, the CRMC Board gave immediate credibility to David Karzon's madcap schemes. Allaire Karzon said:

> At that time Nelson Andrews was president of McClure's [department store] and was a major figure in town. He helped pick the board and filled it with men of stature in town who could negotiate with the Board of Trust of the University as equals, which was essential for them to get that independence. And women, too. He picked superb women.[6]

These board members were savvy enough to realize that although they'd been granted remarkably little authority, in order to persuade others to fall in line, they'd have to behave as if they'd been given enormous power. Former board member Ed Nelson compared those early days to the ingenuity of the bumblebee. "The bee doesn't know that, aerodynamically speaking, it can't fly," he noted.

> Those of us on the Children's Hospital Board were totally unaware that we couldn't fly. If you're not even worried about whether it can be done or not, things somehow get done . . . So we stumbled, threatened, and badgered Vanderbilt.[7]

And, miraculously, they began to establish a hospital.

David Karzon knew he was going to have to finance the project with donations and foundation money, so he started applying for grants to create laboratory space. Lab space is akin to manna for academic physicians, and the pediatric chairman was going to be hiring a lot of new doctors in the near future. Vanderbilt generously offered him ninety-six hundred square feet of shell space, leaving him to figure out how to land the $1.4 million in funds required to build it out. Shortly afterwards, he received a five-hundred-thousand-dollar foundation grant for renovating the donated shell space and purchasing new equipment for the pediatric laboratories.[8] That grant provided both seed money and a psychological boost, fanning the enthusiasm and the faith of his volunteer board.

His next step was to change the ambiance of the pediatric unit. Although great science and great medicine were being practiced on his unit, they were taking place despite near Third World conditions. Libby Werthan remembered a harrowing time when her infant son became extremely ill and stayed at Vanderbilt for over a week. She was allowed to be in the room with him only during brief visiting hours. The corridors on the children's unit were painted a "sick pea green," she recalled.

> It really became terribly obvious to me that something needed to be done. The parents were sleeping in the halls. There were no vending machines. If you had to make a phone call, you had to go to a pay phone. If you didn't have the right change, you were up a creek. It was a very tense situation.

As bad as the circumstances were for her, however, they were far worse for those who didn't live within commuting distance. Werthan continued:

> Because it was a regional hospital, people were coming from out of town. They had their blankets and were sleeping on the floor. There were no sleeper chairs in the rooms, no telephones in the rooms, no place for them to wash up, no place for them to eat or get coffee. It was a really bad situation. It was very primitive.[9]

Once the pediatric unit had metamorphosed into a pediatric "hospital," Karzon could implement changes to bring his unit into the twentieth century. First, he removed the restrictions preventing parents from staying in the rooms with their children. The nurses challenged him, saying, "The children cry when their parents leave!"

"Then encourage the parents to stay!" Karzon retorted. He believed that the pediatric nurses were dedicated caregivers but had never been exposed to alternative approaches. He wanted sleeper chairs in the room so that parents could spend the night and comfort their children, relieving the overworked nursing staff from that chore.

Additionally, he demanded that the hospital dieticians cook food that children might actually eat, instead of feeding them whatever was on the adults' menu. The dieticians protested that separate menus wouldn't be cost effective. Karzon countered that nothing was more wasteful than throwing away all the food on every pediatric tray.

And, he added, children who are starving take longer to recover from their illnesses.[10]

The transformation in pediatric care that was storming through Vanderbilt was indicative of an awareness happening throughout Western medicine in the 1970s, said Stuart Finder. Caregivers were beginning to appreciate that the environment surrounding health delivery was a factor in the speed of a child's recovery. "The existential being," he said, "was viewed as just as important as the physical being."[11]

While all these adjustments were happening at Vanderbilt, the Junior League of Nashville was shaping its own course of destiny. Betty Nelson Burch had assumed the presidency of the League for the 1970–71 term, and Suzanne Woolwine was chair of the Home Board. Both women faced daunting decisions and a split constituency. Several leaders of the organization traveled to New York for a brainstorming session with the National Junior League Association's officers to discuss procedures for a smooth transition. The national group had long believed that the Nashville chapter had held onto the Home for Crippled Children for too many years, which prevented them from investing in other volunteer projects, and they supported the decision for the Nashville Junior League to divest itself of the Home. Headquarters advised the Nashville women to involve as many people as possible in the details so that nobody would feel blindsided.

Back home, the responsibility for setting up and facilitating the public conferences and grievance airings fell on the shoulders of petite, quiet-voiced Betty Nelson Burch.

"She's a little thing, but she's tough as a nickel steak," commented Nelson Andrews.

> And she was able to be a diplomat. There was sort of a cadre of Junior Leaguers who were for [moving the Home to Vanderbilt] and they all took some beatings from fellow Junior Leaguers, from wives of pediatricians, and from pediatricians.[12]

David Karzon attended an open meeting called by the Junior League to solicit public participation in the decision about whether or not to join forces with Vanderbilt. He was amazed as the atmosphere turned angrier and more raucous. Yet Burch stood firm "like Joan of Arc wielding her little, gentle sword, and saying, 'but this is the right thing to do!'"[13]

Suzanne "Suzie" Woolwine was also caught up in the fracas.

Some people felt like we ought to keep going no matter what, even if we had one child left in the building, we ought to keep it open. But I didn't feel that way. I felt that was not a good use of the money and I felt like the children's hospital was part of the growth of this city.[14]

In mid-November, the Junior League of Nashville membership took a vote. The majority opted to close the Home on White Avenue and transfer it to the Children's Regional Medical Center at Vanderbilt. After the announcement, the atmosphere in the room was a mélange of relief, hard feelings, and uncertainty.

Hindsight calls for a philosophic view of events. "The membership was not 100 percent in favor of it," admitted former Junior League president Liza Beazley Lentz. "But the membership has never been 100 percent in favor of anything!"[15]

The newspapers ran announcements about the merger. Jeanne Zerfoss, who had tangled with Amos Christie years before as president of the Junior League in the 1960s, wrote the *Banner's* story. She was also the wife of pediatrician Tommy Zerfoss, who'd vigorously campaigned for a children's hospital. Jeanne Zerfoss was able to reel in Cornelia Ewing, founder of the Junior League of Nashville and now a senior citizen, for a quote. Mrs. Ewing said:

The Junior League is most fortunate to be able to lend financial assistance, moral support, leadership and volunteer efforts toward further establishing such a vitally needed facility as the Children's Regional Medical Center. It puts us in the position of making a community contribution, maintaining our identity as part of this facility, and most important of all, insuring [sic] the care of convalescent children in whose welfare we dedicated ourselves some 48 years ago.[16]

Nelson Andrews told the reporter he was thrilled that the Junior League would be throwing its energies behind the new CRMC. Betty Nelson Burch added that the children would benefit by being placed in a unit with emergency services readily accessible.[17] In the forefront of everyone's minds, but left unsaid, was that the previous year's Palm Sunday Paper Sale had raised over $230,000. Those kinds of six-figure funds would provide a nice annual subsidy to Karzon's pet project. Vanderbilt promised the

Junior League to renovate the Medical Center wing D-3100 into a pediatric convalescent care unit that would contain fourteen beds and a nursing station, and offer nursing utilities, a treatment room, recreation therapy, a playroom, and physical therapy in adjacent pediatric areas. All of those functions and activities would be moved into the Round Wing building upon completion of the new adult hospital.

The plans also called for the state of Tennessee's Department of Mental Health to take over the Home on White Avenue to house the Regional Intervention Project (RIP), an experimental program dealing with the detection and treatment of childhood emotional disorders.

One month later, the Junior League of Nashville and Vanderbilt University entered into a formal agreement to place the Junior League Convalescent Home within the CRMC, which Vanderbilt agreed to have ready for occupancy by August 1, 1971. On that date the League would present the CRMC with a check for two hundred thousand dollars to be used towards defraying building costs and for programs to benefit the new Home's patients. In addition, net income from the Junior League Trust Fund, which then totaled around ninety-one thousand dollars a year, would be donated to the Children's Regional Medical Center to support the care of indigent children on the wing.

The contract read: "The Center will maintain detailed records of expenditures of the fund and make these available for inspection to the League."[18] Vanderbilt, which had never been known for rigorous bookkeeping, would soon learn that the women of the Junior League were dead serious about that particular clause.

Finally, the Junior League agreed to continue the Palm Sunday Paper Sale for another year and then turn over that responsibility to the Medical Center. Before that arrangement had a chance to be tested, however, the Shriners unexpectedly backed out.

For over a decade, the Imperial Council of the national Shriners had looked askance at the Nashville chapter's extraordinary exertion on behalf of a non-Shrine hospital. Over the decades, the relationship between Al Menah Temple and the Junior League had become like a seasoned marriage—meaning it was easier to stay together than to get divorced. On the other hand, the local Shriners retained no similar affection for or loyalty to Vanderbilt. They felt that the behemoth Medical Center had already squeezed them out of the Trust money from the Crippled Children's Home. They could take a hint. The

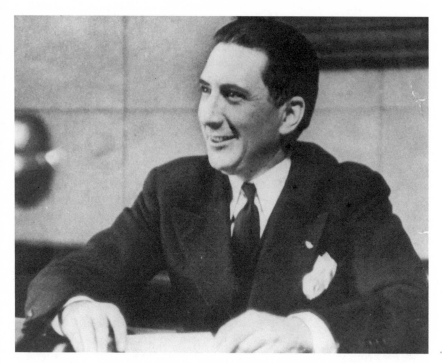

When the Al Menah Shriners backed out of the Palm Sunday Paper Sale, Banner publisher Jimmy Stahlman offered to publish a separate tabloid to benefit the Shrine burn centers.

time had come, they believed, to part ways with the Palm Sunday Paper Sale.

In terms of manpower, this left the organizers of the fund-raiser about six thousand men short. John Seigenthaler was caught in the middle. Shriner Jack Norman had been a lawyer for the *Tennessean* and had helped out Seigenthaler many times over the years. Norman and other Shriner buddies sidled up to the editor, called in a few favors, and asked him to turn the Palm Sunday tabloid over to the Shriners to benefit their burn centers. Seigenthaler refused, knowing that to do so would essentially destroy the credibility the Children's Regional Medical Center was struggling to build and deprive it of a large stash of donated money.

"The Junior League already had me before the Shriners got me and I couldn't go back on my commitment to them," Seigenthaler said. He also added, "It was the first time I'd ever heard the words 'burn center.' I didn't even know they existed."[19]

Fortunately for the Al Menah Temple, Shriner Jimmy Stahlman was cognizant of the burn centers. In January, the *Banner* proclaimed that beginning in October, the Shriners would conduct their own annual paper sale, independent of the Junior League, and the afternoon daily would publish the tabloid.

"As we prepare to continue our efforts in this direction, we wish the young ladies of the Nashville Junior League every success in their new undertaking," Potentate Coleman Hayes said.[20]

With the Vanderbilt arrangement for the Home already forged, Junior League President Betty Nelson Burch thought the most difficult days were behind her—until the Shriners withdrew from the paper sale. She immediately had to switch gears and launch a last-minute campaign to gather five thousand volunteers willing to rise up early on a Sunday in April and fan out to knock on doors across Middle Tennessee.

Burch said, "At first, it was a very scary time. We went and talked to all the civic organizations that had been supporters. I can remember going to forty-one counties and asking them for help."

The Leaguers faced another leviathan challenge in their fundraiser. At that point, no crippled children's room existed at Vanderbilt hospital, much less a devoted convalescent wing for pediatric patients. They would be asking local citizens to donate to a concept, an idea, rather than an existing structure.

"We didn't even have a plaque in the Children's Hospital," Burch said.[21]

Luckily, the Junior League did have a reputation, which counted for quite a bit among Middle Tennesseans. Only a few weeks after the Shriners withdrew, the Civitan Club volunteered its fifteen hundred members to help sell the tabloid.[22] Eight days later, the Nashville chapter of the Frontiers International Club—an African American men's civic organization—stepped forward to cover the North Nashville area for the paper sale.

"We recognize the Junior League people as doing outstanding civic work . . . the work they do is most unselfish," said Alfred C. Galloway, chairman of Frontiers's executive committee. "This program they have sponsored in the past deserves assistances [*sic*] from all community service organizations."[23]

Once the Frontiersmen joined in the effort, civic groups from across the area stepped up. Although the number of volunteers fell short of five thousand, absent the heft of the Shrine organization, many people who had never before participated in the Palm Sunday Paper Sale responded to the League's call. In the end, the sale raised well over one hundred thousand dollars that first year without the Shriners—about half of what it had earned in previous years, but still a welcomed infusion of money for the CRMC.

On another note, the Frontiers's involvement signaled something else much more subtle, yet truly profound. A decade earlier, the Junior League, which had no African Americans among its membership, had quietly and resolutely integrated the Home for Crippled Children. When the Frontiersmen stepped forward to help out the League, they just as quietly and resolutely were letting them know that they had noticed.

One of the greatest hurdles faced both by David Karzon and the Junior League was enlightening the public on the strategy behind the Children's Regional Medical Center. The hospital was a patchwork, scattered on various floors and in several buildings throughout Vanderbilt Hospital—including the acute care pediatric wards, the pediatric surgical unit, the pediatric intensive care unit, the newborn nursery, the newborn intensive care unit, the pediatric ambulatory unit, and the specialized diagnostic and research pediatric laboratories. David Karzon agreed to a series of interviews to explain his theory defining a hospital-within-a-hospital.

> . . . The Children's Hospital is more than geography, more than a place . . . It consists of all those areas that care for children in Vanderbilt University Hospital . . . The Children's Hospital is not bricks and mortar, it is a way of approaching children's medical needs.[24]

Karzon's new-fangled concept was difficult for Nashvillians to grasp. Even worse, it became a laughingstock for academic physicians who worked in freestanding children's hospitals around the country, said Ian Burr, who joined the faculty in 1971 as a pediatric endocrinologist. "People were rather nasty at times," he remembered. "They said, 'You don't really have a children's hospital!'—which we didn't. They said, 'It's a marketing ploy and you're conning the public!'"

But, Burr added:

> Having [the CRMC] in the hospital was not a bad idea financially, at least to start with. In fact, it was a good idea. And certainly it was a good idea in terms of getting the thought of a children's hospital in people's minds. Our critics were right—it was great marketing.[25]

This calculated game of who's conning whom continued until the hospital-within-a-hospital gained traction in the local community. Part of the unique culture of Nashville is that its citizens are comfortable choosing a path of nonconformity, and they don't particularly care if outsiders are laughing at them. Actually, in testament to poetic justice, over the course of the years, scores of pediatricians and hospital administrators visited Vanderbilt Children's Hospital to find out how to successfully create a similar configuration in their own medical centers.

While the CRMC was still in its formative stages, however, David Karzon suffered some bruises but held firm to his strategy—and his maverick board faithfully backed him up.

In the early 1970s, two things occurred that added weight to the pediatric hospital's legitimacy—the Junior League finally moved its Home for Crippled Children over to Vanderbilt, and a plucky group of CRMC board members spun off into an ad hoc committee devoted strictly to fund-raising. Calling themselves the Friends of Children's Hospital, these women were industrious, creative, and charmingly audacious.

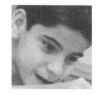

Friends Arrive on the Scene | 15

"[The Friends of the Children's Hospital] was an outlaw board. It had no legal standing. We just created ourselves. It was a matter of some community people realizing that there was a need and having the will to make it happen out of thin air."

—Libby Werthan,
first president of Friends of the Children's Hospital

"We were flying 'nekkid.'"

—Carole Nelson,
first treasurer of Friends of the Children's Hospital

A ugust 1, 1971, marked the end of a long, gut-wrenching journey by the Junior League of Nashville. On that bitter-sweet day, a skeleton crew of personnel loaded up the four patients residing at the Home for Crippled Children and transported them by station wagon over to Vanderbilt Hospital. League member Judy Haworth, director of the Home, led the way in her car. After seeing the children safely admitted into their rooms at Vanderbilt, "she returned to 2400 White Avenue, secured the premises, and drove home 'crying all the way.'"[1]

Suzie Woolwine was the Home Board chair at the time. Faced with so many conflicting feelings when the day finally arrived, she chose not to take part in actually moving the children.

She explained:

I had a big emotional tie to the Junior League Home, because I'd done so much of my volunteer work there. And I loved it. I loved the

179

people who worked there. They were just top-notch. It was like a home. The dietician, the occupational therapist, the physical therapist, everybody, they all got along well together. It was just a happy place to be.

Woolwine waited until she knew the children were already on the unit, sucked up her courage, and drove over to check on everyone. The admission process went smoothly and quickly, she recalled. The children were going to be okay.[2] Also on that day, the League officially disbanded the position of Home Board chair. The ladies of the Junior League tenderly understood that a storied era in Nashville's history had just come to an end.

To ensure an amicable dialogue, Nelson Andrews opened positions on the CRMC Board for Junior League representatives to serve as liaisons between the organization and the hospital. Andrews's act essentially unlocked the floodgates. These early liaisons from the Junior League barreled onto the board with unflappable grit and a certainty of purpose.

One of these representatives was Irene Wills, whose father-in-law Jesse Wills had served on the Children's Hospital Board. Although Vanderbilt was considered off-limits by many of Nashville's affluent families, the Willses believed in and trusted the institution, which is why Irene chose to give birth to her children there. Tragically, her second son, also named Jesse Wills, was born with a heart defect. After a raft of surgeries, tests, and surgical revisions at Vanderbilt, and later by famed cardiac surgeon Dr. Denton Cooley at Texas Children's Hospital in Houston, little Jesse died at age two.

"When I came back [from Houston] I said I'm going to make things better in Nashville," Irene recalled. "That's why I got on a crusade to make the hospital better."[3]

When Jesse died, Irene was already seven months pregnant with her third son, Morgan. In early April 1968, she woke up and told her husband that the baby was coming and they'd better to rush to the hospital. Driving down West End Avenue at a speedy clip, they passed Centennial Park and noticed with alarm that the park was bustling with ominous commotion. The National Guard had stationed armored tanks inside the city of Nashville. Dr. Martin Luther King had been shot and killed a few nights before in Memphis, sparking demonstrations and disturbances all across the country. Nashville's mayor was preparing for a race riot.

Although Wills gave birth to her son by 5:00 AM, the residents wouldn't allow her to go up to her hospital room, nor would they bring her the baby. Finally, at eleven o'clock that morning she was near hysterics, worried that something was wrong with her child. A bedraggled nurse appeared a short time later, carrying Irene's healthy baby boy into the room. "We're so sorry," said the nurse. "We're just so short of help. None of the black nurses came in today."[4]

The race riot never happened. Instead Nashvillians convened in Centennial Park and grieved over the loss of King, while a few blocks away Irene Wills comforted and nurtured her newborn son.

The other Junior League representative named to the CRMC Board was Linda Christie Williams (now Moynihan), the daughter of Amos Christie. Although her father had obstinately opposed the construction of a children's hospital at Vanderbilt, Williams held a personal stake in the outcome. Despite objections from some, the CRMC was being created and she, probably more than any single person in Nashville, wanted to see it thrive. After all, her father's legacy depended on the continued success of Vanderbilt pediatrics.

One of the first things Williams did when she took her seat on the board was to propose that the CRMC establish a separate ad hoc committee for fund-raising, to be called the Friends of the Children's Hospital. Such a group would serve as a mechanism for attracting large amounts of individual giving to the children's center.[5]

Karzon's initial proposal to the Vanderbilt Board of Trust had actually included a request that a Children's Fund be set up for charitable giving to the CRMC. He was not quite certain what the women were cooking up with the Friends proposition, but he went along anyway, aware that he needed the support of all the Junior Leaguers he could muster. What they had in mind, as it turned out, was to bring a "woman's touch"[7] into the growth and development of the Children's Hospital at Vanderbilt.

Beyond that, however, Williams and fellow board member Peggy Steine recognized that they'd been given an unprecedented opportunity to unify the community through the Friends organization. For her part, Williams particularly wanted to bring the Jewish and Christian communities together. "I'd put up a number of people for membership in the Junior League over the years and I know the only reason they didn't get in was because they were Jewish," she said. "And it just made me so mad, because there was miraculous talent there."[7]

So, Williams asked Peggy Steine, a leader in local Jewish circles, to figure out the best person—who also happened to be Jewish—to serve as the Friends' first president. Peggy Steine was sure that Libby Werthan was the right woman for the job.

"All of a sudden it started snowballing," recalled Williams, who'd been appointed second vice president and paper sales chair.

When it first started, every member of Friends was also an officer. Dean Reeves was corresponding secretary; Jan Riven (another Jewish member) became recording secretary; Carole Nelson moved from the Junior League to assume the role of treasurer; Mary Henderson, who had recently relocated to Nashville from Texas, was named president-elect; and Berenice Denton was first vice president.

To broaden the Friends Board even further, Peggy Steine, Libby Werthan, and Linda Williams hoped to convince an African American to join them. Joan Bahner agreed to become the parliamentarian of the fledgling organization. A graduate of Fisk University, mother of four children, and the wife of local pediatrician Roderick Bahner, Joan felt duty-bound to volunteer wherever she could. The Werthan and the Bahner children attended Peabody Demonstration School (now University School of Nashville) together. Bahner knew she could make important inroads—and since Vanderbilt was just across the street from her children's school, accepting a spot on the Friends Board seemed like an efficient starting point.

Joan Bahner recalled:

> I was eager to help, eager to represent my people. I would say yes to about any task of volunteerism that was brought before me. There were plenty of African American women much brighter than me, probably with a lot better ideas than I had. But I just happened to be the one with the gumption and the moxie to get out there and do.

Like a clarion call, Bahner's role on the Friends Board got the attention of people across the city. The Children's Hospital was to be a place for everybody. On the other hand, not everyone in Nashville's upscale African American society was impressed. One of Bahner's friends referred to her as "Miss Vanderbilt," which was not intended to be a compliment.

"It was really a kind of put-down," Bahner said. "But I was so energized, I just put on blinders and kept going."[8]

The Friends enjoyed their renegade status. "It was an outlaw board," explained Libby Werthan. "It had no legal standing. We just created ourselves. It was a matter of some community people realizing that there was a need and having the will to make it happen out of thin air."[9]

They wrote a set of bylaws and prayed none of the higher-ups would question their authority to do that. "We were flying 'nekkid,'" admitted Carole Nelson.

One of the first tasks this dynamic gang of eight pursued was to formulate an identity, including a logo. When they were discussing how best to represent the new hospital, Carole Nelson took out an old check, flipped it over, and penciled in a rudimentary sketch of two stick figures holding hands.

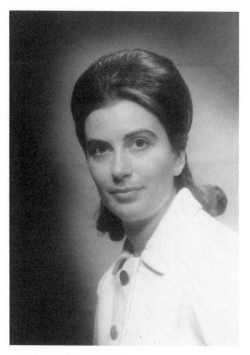

Libby Werthan served as the first president of the Friends of the Children's Hospital at Vanderbilt. The goal of Friends was not only to raise money for the hospital, but also to unite various factions of the community.

"This is what it needs to be," she announced.[10]

From that crude drawing, Dean Reeves fashioned the sketch to look like cutout paper dolls, which still stands as the logo for Vanderbilt Children's Hospital today. For years, the Friends fought "tooth and toenail" to prevent some slick marketing firm from changing the logo into a more sophisticated image. In keeping with the fashion palette of the '70s, they selected the color scheme for their stationary and other materials to be an orange logo on a yellow background. (In time, the color scheme morphed into a red logo on a white background. The women weren't nearly as adamant about the color scheme issue.)

Because pediatric rooms were strewn around the old Vanderbilt Hospital, the ladies cut the paper doll logos out of contact paper, then

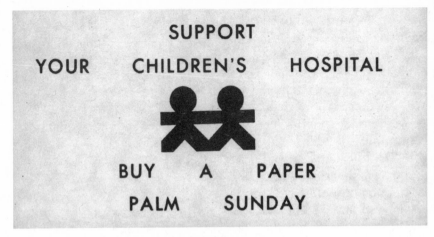

In order to establish an identity for the hospital-within-a-hospital, the Friends created the children-holding-hands logo and put it wherever children were being treated at Vanderbilt.

went around the building taping them on the doors in the Round Wing and down any hall where children were located.

"We had to have some identifier," said Linda Williams. "That's all we had to show."[11]

Within the first year of existence, the Friends Board wrote a catchy musical jingle that appeared in all their radio and public service announcements, they brought in clowns and celebrities to perform for the children, and they changed the name of the hospital.

In an effort to be all-inclusive, Vanderbilt had arrived at a name— Children's Regional Medical Center—which was so awkward and forgettable that it became almost impossible to use for fund-raising. "Nobody could understand what it was, and the doctors themselves called it the 'pediatric unit,'" said Alice Hooker, who would soon join the Friends Board. "So right then I really got agitated and said that it had to have a name change."[12]

By approval of the hospital board, the Children's Regional Medical Center became the Children's Hospital at Vanderbilt University.

The next item on the agenda was for the women of Friends to convince Vanderbilt to let them have their own interest-bearing account. Carole Nelson and Libby Werthan approached Vanderbilt Medical Center's financial officer, Paul Gazzerro. "He was a very intimidating gentleman," Nelson recalled. "He reminded me of Kojak. He had a bald head, and intense, fierce eyes. When Libby and

I met with him he informed us that under no circumstances would he let us have an interest-bearing account."

That was the wrong answer. Every week, Carole Nelson steeled herself and met with Gazzerro, insisting that he allow them to set up such an account. Every week, Gazzerro became angrier, yelled louder, and turned them down more ferociously. Nelson was almost sick to her stomach after she left his office, but she kept going back. "All we are is a pediatric wing and we need a way to have an identity," she told him. "We cannot have it if we don't have financial clout. And we are starting from so far behind that we have to have this!"

Eventually, she outlasted him and Gazzerro granted the Friends permission to control their own separate account. Nelson had been right. That account gave the Friends organizational clout and bargaining power. They could access that money for projects they thought were important without having to go through cumbersome university channels. The money they raised became theirs.

The Friends of the Children's Hospital grew like wildfire. From a band of eight desperados, the organization bloomed to nearly three hundred members by the end of the first year. They set up a tier of membership levels: Founding members gave at $300; Life members at $150; Mr. & Mrs. at $10; Single at $5; and Regional at $2.[13] People of Middle Tennessee rallied in support and donated over $20,000 to the fund.

The Friends embarked on a variety of projects. They had the patients in the Children's Hospital draw pictures for Christmas tags and later, Christmas cards, which were sold as a fund-raiser during the holiday season—and as a year-end reminder to donors. The women purchased diapers for indigent babies and clothes for pediatric patients who only had hospital pajamas to wear. They hired a Child Life Specialist to engage the children in play therapy and help prepare them psychologically for surgery. They insisted that emergency physicians set aside two special rooms for children in the Emergency Room, which the Friends group decorated with colorful wallpaper and welcoming decor. The newspapers and radio stations could hardly run enough stories mentioning the good deeds by the Friends of Children's Hospital at Vanderbilt.

This created its own set of internal issues within the Medical Center. Physicians in other specialties grew jealous that Children's Hospital was soaking up all the media attention and most of the charitable contributions. A geriatrician approached Carole Nelson

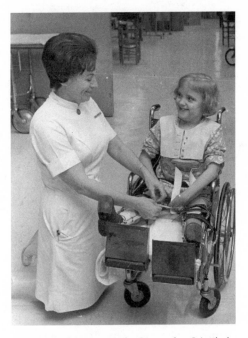

Many employees at the Home for Crippled Children, including head nurse Christine Branch, transferred to the new Junior League Home Unit at Children's Regional Medical Center.

asking, "Why can't I have a hospital for old people?" Cardiologists demanded that they needed a hospital for heart patients. Nephrologists questioned why there was no "Friends of Kidney Disease" out raising money for them. They wondered why David Karzon should be the only Vanderbilt doctor with an adoring entourage of women funneling money his way. When pediatrics secured precious in-house real estate for a playroom— deemed a safe haven for patients where doctors and staff members were not allowed to perform any medical procedures—other faculty members blew a gasket.

"That was a bitter, bitter battle," Nelson recalled.

Before closing the Home on White Avenue, the League had arranged for as many of the employees as were interested to transfer their jobs over to Vanderbilt. Christine Branch was a registered nurse at the Home who chose to continue working on the Junior League Home Unit. At that time the admissions criteria for the Home Unit included the following:

1. no severely ill patient should be admitted;
2. postoperative patients must be essentially well (frequent IVs or intensive nursing not needed);
3. patients do not go directly into surgery or come directly out of surgery.[14]

In other words, the idea was for the Junior League Home Unit to serve exclusively as a convalescence area from non-life-threatening illnesses. Such are the best-laid plans. In the beginning, the reality proved much more complicated than that.

Construction continued on the Children's Hospital within the hospital. In January 1972, the wing for the Junior League Home Unit was finally completed and was formally dedicated the next month. The rooms were crisp and sparkling and the ancillary services were first-rate.

Almost immediately, David Karzon faced unexpected problems. First, the regular pediatric rooms looked sterile and shabby compared to those on the Home Unit. Since it was nicer and had a full array of therapists and specialists at the patients' disposal, physicians began finagling to get their patients onto the Home Unit, whether or not they met the stated criteria. The nursing staff of the ward protested, arguing that they were not trained to deal with the types of cases that were being admitted there. Also, whenever the regular pediatric unit became full, the admitting officers simply ignored the parameters and automatically sent children onto the Home Unit if beds were available. In short order, tensions began to boil.

Karzon realized he was going to have to spiff up all of pediatrics. At the Children's Hospital Board meeting, he told the members that the projected cost of renovating the other wings, D-3200 and S-3300, into cheerful, bright, modern areas would be "staggering"—somewhere in excess of $175,000, not even counting the loss of patient income during the renovation period. The board, in turn, argued that it ought to be the responsibility of Vanderbilt Hospital, not the CRMC board, to cover those renovation expenses.[15] Karzon, however, would not let the matter drop.

Meanwhile, Linda Williams's efforts to unify the various sectors of Nashville society had worked all too well. If the Junior League was powerful beforehand, it became titanic when it joined forces with the officers of Friends. Libby Werthan lassoed Vanderbilt trustees Pat Wilson and Tom Kennedy. After a tour of the facilities and a long conversation with them over lunch, Werthan fired off a letter on behalf of herself, Friends members Linda Christie Williams and Mary Henderson, and Children's Hospital board members and Junior Leaguers Irene Wills, Mary Stumb, and Peggy Warner.

"The Children's Hospital finds itself at a crossroads," Werthan told the trustees. "It has the potential of becoming not only an outstanding regional center, but one of national and international acclaim—or, it can backslide into just another mediocre hospital."[16]

She then listed the points that favored its leaning towards greatness, such as an outstanding staff of doctors and programs, fine laboratory facilities, and the financial and moral support of the surrounding community.

Werthan went on to say that in spite of these strengths, the Children's Hospital stood to "lose it all" due to the following weaknesses.

The present facilities are inadequate, antiquated, demoralizing and dehumanizing.

Examples—(a) There are not enough bathrooms (in some instances sick children must walk through other sick children's rooms to get to the bathroom). (b) Parents must be considered as well as children in a Children's Hospital. They sometimes stay a week at a time with no shower facilities and poor bathroom facilities. (c) There is practically no storage area for patients and parents, creating a condition of constant clutter in the rooms. (d) Minimum health standards are not always adhered to—until recently body wastes were being collected and emptied in the same room as the ice machine. (e) Many pediatricians shy away from the Children's Hospital, even though they know the medical care is better, simply because they don't want to listen to parents complain (there are a number of medical facilities available in Nashville that are modern, clean and comfortable). (f) Because parents generally stay with their children and often for long periods of time, food is being brought into the hospital (although strongly discouraged) that, along with poor housekeeping, creates a problem with roaches and other insects. (g) The window air conditioners function in such a way that they blow right on the child next to the window and the child across the room swelters when the curtain is drawn between the beds.

"We feel that we are in great danger of losing community support if the community does not see tangible evidence of improvement in the near future," she concluded.[17]

The end result of all this hectoring by the concerned ladies of the city was that the sleeping Medical Center dinosaur began to awaken and slowly acknowledge that enhancements could be made even while blueprints for a new hospital were still being drawn. In that vein, the Friends initiated "Operation Facelift," a citywide volunteer effort where local civic groups donated time to spruce up individual rooms in the hospital that served children.

As if the interactions with the Friends weren't enough for the Medical Center, in order to stay true to the rules of the Trust, the Junior League demanded from Vanderbilt a detailed account of how the hospital was spending every dime of their donations. League President Peggy Warner chose to play tough. After contributing $161,276.61 to the Home Unit (beyond the initial $200,000), Warner withheld further payment, citing a clause in their contract: "The Center will maintain detailed records of expenditures of the fund and make these available for inspection by the League." Until they saw accounting records, the League refused to further consider any requests by Vanderbilt for funds to renovate the other pediatric areas.

"Financial statements covering the Junior League endowment expenditures . . . are a 'must' as far as we are concerned," Warner wrote. "Certainly the Executive Board of the Children's Hospital should have an up-to-date accounting of the Children's Fund before we seek the financial support of the people of this region on Palm Sunday."[18]

For the first time in its history, Vanderbilt's pediatric department had to develop operational procedures for giving financial reports to an outside entity. Warner's letter was a jolt. Suddenly, the Medical Center had to be vigilant in keeping track of its income and expenditures. A month later, Paul Gazzerro sent the League its requested financial statement of accounting and promised that in the future he would deliver further reports to the League on a monthly basis.[19]

Although David Karzon had never been a part of the socially elite crowd growing up, he was acutely aware of the sway they wielded and was wise enough to make them feel appreciated. From the starting bell, the alumnae of the Delta Delta Delta sorority at Vanderbilt took on the Children's Hospital as a worthy cause. In 1970, they initiated the Eve of Janus New Year's Eve Ball, "a glittering black-tie affair,"[20] to benefit Karzon's vision for pediatric health care. The first Eve of Janus Ball went so swimmingly that the Tri-Delts made it a yearly event, appealing to the exclusivity of the occasion. Local businesses sponsored a coed participant, donating one hundred dollars towards the Children's Fund for that privilege. Wrote Susan Brandau of the *Tennessean*, "A highlight of the glittering affair will be the presentation . . . of 25 Nashville girls representing the 'Signs of the Times' and costumed to represent the local business firms which sponsor them. These girls, chosen by secret committee, are all college students and members of various sororities."[21] Over the years, the Tri-Delts raised huge sums of money for the Children's Hospital.

On the other side of the equation, much of the early fund-raising was directed at the general public, the people for whom a nearby children's hospital would become a beacon. When the Junior League of Nashville bequeathed the Palm Sunday Paper Sale to the Friends of Children's Hospital, individuals from all walks of life stepped up to help in this massive undertaking.[22] Joanne Nairon recounted sitting in her office at the Friends headquarters when William Ross, an employee with the campus mail service, came in to see her. Ross had worked at Vanderbilt since 1951 as a chauffeur for Chancellor Branscomb and various trustees and as a jack-of-all-trades in the administration offices. He was known by many of the pediatric patients as "Sweet William," a stage name he used in *The Bozo Show* and when he'd perform his sleight-of-hand act in the schools and for hospitalized children.[23]

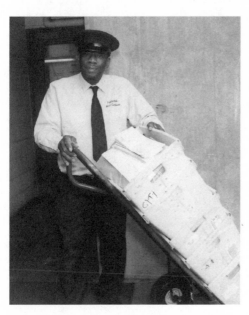

Once the Palm Sunday Paper Sale moved over to Vanderbilt, mail clerk William Ross made it a point to be the first person to donate each year for the next twenty-five years.

Early in the morning on the first day of the Friends' paper sale, William Ross approached Joanne Nairon and pulled a bill from his pocket. "I want to be the first one to give to the Children's Hospital," he said.

Every year after that, until the door-to-door Palm Sunday Paper Sale ended in the late 1990s, William Ross made it a point to donate the first dollar. His contribution became an unheralded annual tradition, a good luck charm for the launching of the fund-raiser each spring.[24]

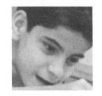

Growth Spurt | 16

"You know what's expected of you. You're expected to build a clinical program, do research, publish, and start a training program."

**—Dr. David Karzon's directive
to the young subspecialists he hired as pediatric division chiefs**

While external forces were implanting new ideas into Vanderbilt University Medical Center, internal factors were also changing the dynamics of the practice of pediatric medicine. The Neonatal Intensive Care Unit, under the command of Mildred Stahlman, had already sown the seeds of progress. After David Karzon took over the controls of the pediatrics department, those seeds began to blossom and mature.

In the early 1970s, Stahlman expanded the scope of the NICU by establishing a regional transport system for bringing premature infants to the hospital. The NICU staff and faculty had become increasingly angry and frustrated as a continuous stream of babies reached Vanderbilt Hospital dead on arrival. The tipping point came when Vanderbilt received in one traumatic day three babies, all dead on arrival; what's more, all of them had traveled a long distance to get there. Stahlman recalled:

> They came from a hospital that was unable to manage them, that had no ability to stabilize them. The nursing care was inadequate. They had no care in the hour or hour-and-a-half it took them to get here. And they arrived on our doorstep either dead or dying. . . .

191

With the help of people in Memphis and Knoxville we went to
the state and said, "This is intolerable! It's not only bad medicine, it's
bad politics!"[1]

Stahlman, in conjunction with Dr. Frank H. Boehm, who was
recently appointed to head up the division of Maternal-Fetal
Medicine, first began working with the state to improve the outcome
of complicated pregnancies. During those years, if a premature child
were born in an outlying hospital, the doctors would simply wait to
see if the baby survived birth and then call Vanderbilt. Critically ill
infants would be placed into an ambulance, with little or no nursing
care, and by the time they got to the hospital they'd be cold or in
shock. As a remedy, Stahlman and Boehm launched a program for
maternal transports. As many premature babies as possible would
arrive at Vanderbilt still in utero and were delivered there with immediate access to the facilities of the intensive care unit while the mother
was cared for by the obstetrics team.[2]

Adding to the maternal-fetal program in 1972, Vanderbilt's NICU
physicians received a grant from the Regional Appalachian Medical
Program to construct and operate a transport unit for newborns. One
of Stahlman's fellows, Dr. Angela Skelton, disliked working in the
animal lab, so Stahlman gave her the responsibility of suiting up an
appropriate vehicle and organizing the transport system. Skelton
bought a "step van," or in less elegant terms, an old bread truck. She
had Vanderbilt medical instrumentation employees install open bed
warmers, ventilators, and monitoring equipment into the van.

In honor of Angela Skelton, said Robert Cotton, "the instrumentation guy putting the transport truck together didn't ask anybody,
but painted the name 'ANGEL' on the side of the vehicle."[3]

Thus was born the Angel I emergency transport system, which in
its first year served 295 patients from the surrounding area.[4] Since
then, generations of Angel transport vehicles have carried thousands
of critically ill children to Vanderbilt's intensive care units and emergency rooms. In the early 1970s, as a result of Angel I, the NICU
census skyrocketed. The transportation of babies in distress became a
hallmark of Vanderbilt Medical Center.

One day, however, a neonatal nurse pointed out to the officers of
the Friends organization that an unforeseen dilemma had arisen. The
mothers from outlying areas being served by Angel I had trouble
bonding with their babies. Often the infants had been snatched from

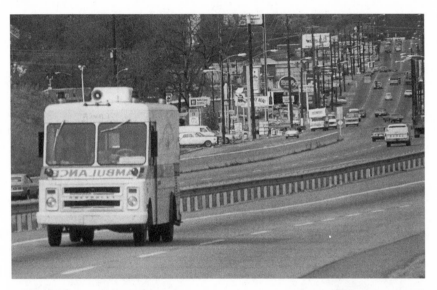

The NICU team converted an old bread truck into the Angel ambulance for trans-porting premature infants to the NICU.

the mother immediately after birth, hauled off to Vanderbilt, and had remained there for weeks or months. Many rural women, too poor to make the journey to Nashville, hardly had a chance to see their little ones before they were whisked away. So when the baby finally was well enough to return home to the mother, they acted like strangers. Neither the parent nor the child experienced any kind of unique, mother-child connection.

The Friends came up with a solution. The organization purchased an expensive camera, took photos of the newborn being cared for by the Vanderbilt team, and kept track of the baby's progress. Carole Nelson said:

> We would get pictures of these babies back to the mother so she could see her child and feel like she was bonding with it. This was when the Friends had very little money. But, gosh, I was proud of that. If that didn't touch you, nothing will.[5]

Stahlman also launched a personal campaign to reform the state's health insurance policies. At that time, a child would not be covered until after he or she was twelve to fourteen days old. Stahlman went to several successive Tennessee governors asking, "Why is a baby not

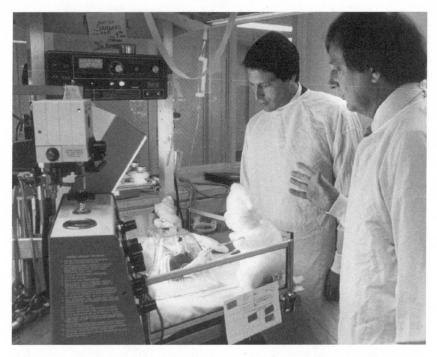

The Angel infant transport system and the Vanderbilt NICU were so acclaimed that politicians, such as Representative Al Gore Jr. (left), came by to tour the facility and discuss issues with NICU physician Dr. Robert Cotton (right).

a person until he's twelve days old and deserves insurance?"[6] She gave slide shows to the state legislature and vehemently argued against the policy. Finally, in 1974, the legislature changed the rules of the program.[7]

During the same time frame when Mildred Stahlman was addressing the pressing issues of neonatology, others began focusing attention on similar needs for children beyond the NICU, which also spurred the expansion of Vanderbilt pediatrics. The primary catalyst for that expansion, borne out of one family's personal tragedy, was the establishment of the Pediatric Intensive Care Unit (PICU).

Although she'd been born in a normal, full-term delivery, Mollie Wilkerson Cook was not a healthy baby. On May 8, 1967, at the age of six weeks, she died of a rare heart defect, despite the best efforts of hospital personnel to save her. In honor of little Mollie, her grandparents, Mr. and Mrs. Charles Cook, and her parents, Mr. and Mrs.

William Cook, approached Vanderbilt about building a special unit for children with severe cardiovascular disease, the PICU.

Until the creation of the PICU, young patients requiring intensive care were simply placed in individual rooms next to the nurses' station. Hospital staff would move all the clumsy paraphernalia—ventilators, tanks, and monitoring devices—in and out of the patients' rooms as needed.[8] Also, the children needing intensive care were placed into rooms with adults in similar straits.

"Mr. [Charles] Cook was horrified when he came into the hospital and saw his tiny little granddaughter surrounded by adults who had been in car wrecks or were dying of heart attacks," Mollie's mother, Jean Cook, recalled. "In 1967, there was no special wing anywhere in Nashville specifically for children who were critically ill or recovering from operations."[9]

The Cooks initially agreed to contribute twenty-five thousand dollars towards the PICU over a five-year period. Instead, they donated that amount within two years, and within five years, had raised over one hundred thousand dollars in total gifts[10]—seventy-seven thousand from the Cook family; twenty-two thousand dollars from the Wills family (Jesse Sr. and Ridley) in memory of Jesse Wills III, who had also died from cardiovascular disease; five thousand dollars from banker and chairman of the Vanderbilt Board of Trust,

The Friends of Children's Hospital purchased a camera so that mothers could bond with their premature infants who were in the NICU. Photo by Jimmy Ellis, Tennessean.

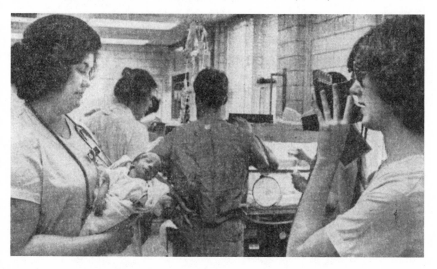

Sam Fleming; and the rest from various other friends of the family. In September 1969, Vanderbilt's first PICU opened with four beds in two adjacent rooms on the third floor of the Round Wing of Vanderbilt University Hospital.[11]

"When my father and I started out on this project to create a PICU at Vanderbilt, I don't think either one of us realized the long-term significance of what we were doing," said Bill Cook, Mollie's father. "We knew a sea change was coming in medicine, but it took us years to understand the vital part the PICU would play in the growth of Children's Hospital."[12]

As far as the construction details, Karzon turned them over to the one person in the hospital with expertise in starting an intensive care unit—Mildred Stahlman. While the Cooks stayed on the outside raising money, Stahlman made sure that the right equipment was acquired and installed.

Vanderbilt's scrawny little PICU would ultimately spark a chain reaction within local pediatrics. First, the PICU was specialized for only

In 1969, Bill Cook and his family underwrote the creation of a Pediatric Intensive Care Unit at Vanderbilt in memory of his daughter, Mollie Wilkerson Cook.

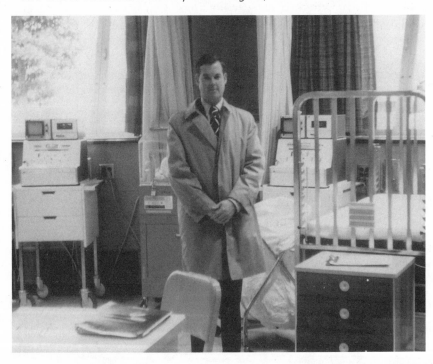

those children needing constant monitoring, which meant it primarily served postoperative patients. The acutely and severely ill child still had no place to go in Vanderbilt Hospital. Within a year, however, additional funding for the PICU enabled the creation of two isolation rooms for children with contagious diseases and for those whose immune systems had been compromised by diseases such as cancer.[13]

Because all of the machines needed in each room took up so much space, parents had no place to stay while their children were being treated in the unit—other than the waiting rooms, which were in a condition that could only be called "disgusting."[14] Shortly, the Friends began raising money to enhance the waiting room environment, including adding reclining chairs for exhausted parents wanting to take a momentary break.

Perhaps most important, the existence of the PICU meant that Karzon had to hire physicians specifically trained to handle those caseloads. The unit created a sudden demand at Vanderbilt for a pediatric surgeon who could perform the intricate life-or-death operations on sick children as well as a pediatric cardiologist who could perform delicate heart procedures and monitor the progress of these children. Any other department chairman might have looked into the crystal ball and been overwhelmed. David Karzon instead saw an unprecedented chance to build a program from the ground up. He began shopping the academic marketplace for recruits.

Immediately, he was confronted with a harsh reality. Having originally intended and attempted to lure seasoned physicians to Vanderbilt, he soon realized he couldn't offer them either the resources or the wages that made it worth the risk to move. Once again, Karzon regrouped and reformulated his plan, this time focusing on energetic young guns—rising stars with several research publications under their belts, but whose enthusiasm vastly outweighed their experience. He began going after youthful physicians, mostly those in their early to mid-thirties, who stood undaunted by the neophyte facilities at Vanderbilt's Children's Hospital, and who were too fresh in their careers to command big salaries. He sought visionaries unafraid of launching into a trial-by-fire learning curve.

Karzon couldn't offer them a lot of money, but he could promise them a golden opportunity to define their subspecialties; in effect, to sculpt and mold a medical field as it was unfolding. He enticed them to come to Vanderbilt by holding up a blank canvas and encouraging

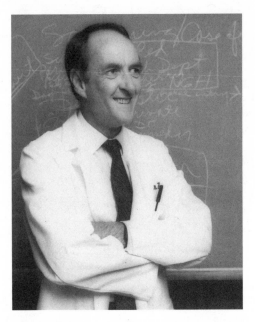

Dr. Ian Burr.

them to test out their ideas. By the end of his tenure, Karzon had slowly and methodically hired a faculty of young, excellent subspecialists, many of them pioneers in pediatric academic research, and many of whom remained at Vanderbilt for the rest of their medical careers.

The first wave of newly hired physicians arrived in Nashville like a band of soldiers. Ian Burr, who received his medical training in his native country of Australia, joined Vanderbilt in January 1971, as the chief of the division of pediatric endocrinology. Although he also had offers from Harvard, Duke, and the University of California at San Francisco, Burr cast his lot with Vanderbilt.

"Vanderbilt at that time, believe it or not, even though it was not nearly as high up on the hierarchy as those others, had the best endocrine program in the country by far," he said.

He added that he was "somewhat shocked" when he first saw the cobbled-together hospital-within-a-hospital, but he was attracted by the high academic standard David Karzon had set for the place. Burr could feel that Vanderbilt was on the upswing—catching up to the rest of the world perhaps, but heading in the right direction.[15]

Another crucial component of Karzon's scheme was to develop the relatively new field of pediatric cardiology. He had already tabbed Dr. Thomas Graham as a potential candidate, even though Graham had only recently completed his fellowship and was working at Duke University Hospital. On his first visit to the campus, Graham recalled, he was in the air flying to Nashville at the exact moment that astronaut Neil Armstrong took a giant leap for mankind by setting foot on the moon. After Graham toured the Children's Hospital at Vanderbilt, he informed Karzon that he simply wasn't ready to take on such a monumental task. Instead he returned to Duke. Two years later, Karzon called again and now he had a new lure: a PICU for treating the most complicated cardiovascular cases. This time Graham was feeling more secure and "excited about the opportunity to develop something from scratch."

Graham said that Karzon was too busy to micromanage his division chiefs. Instead he told them, "You know what's expected of you. You're expected to build a clinical program, do research, publish, and start a training program."[16]

At the same time that he was building the medicine subspecialties, Karzon was aware that he could not truly revolutionize child health care without the assistance of an eager cadre of pediatric surgeons. James O'Neill had undergone his residency training at Vanderbilt in pediatric surgery and later had taken a junior faculty position at Louisiana State University Medical Center in New Orleans (commuting between LSU and Tulane Hospitals). Karzon teamed up with Surgery Chairman William Scott and Orthopedics Chairman William Hillman to convince the young O'Neill to assume the mantle of chief of pediatric surgery at Vanderbilt. Shortly afterwards, Hillman died suddenly at the age of forty-nine, but O'Neill had already decided to gamble and make the transition to Vanderbilt.

Dr. Thomas Graham with patient.

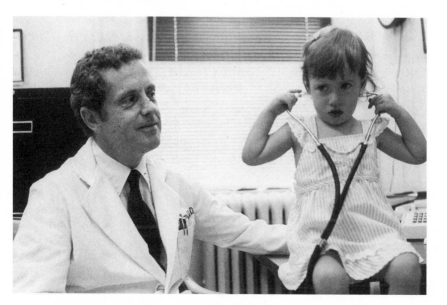

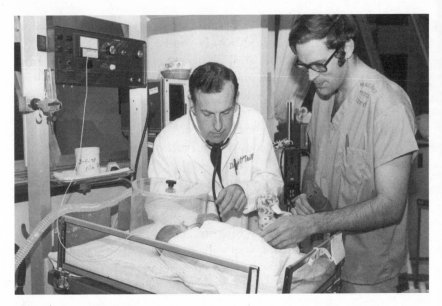

Dr. James O'Neill (left).

In addition, other subspecialties were also ramping up. In 1971 alone, Dr. Harvey Bender joined the faculty in cardiothoracic surgery for both children and adults; Dr. Paul Griffin in children's orthopedic surgery; Dr. Henry Coppolillo in child psychiatry; Dr. Paul Gomez in the outpatient department and the cystic fibrosis clinic; and Dr. Nancie Schweikert in the developmental evaluation clinic. A year later, William Altemeier became chief of pediatrics at Nashville General and Dr. Gerald Atwood joined Tom Graham in pediatric cardiology, followed by Dr. Harold Green in pediatric gastroenterology and Dr. Peter Wright in pediatric infectious diseases.[17]

In other words, the pediatric and surgical faculties experienced a grand explosion. Under Amos Christie, the majority of the pediatrics faculty had graduated from Vanderbilt Medical School.[18] David Karzon, however, selected people from all over the globe. They brought to the table a variety of medical experiences and an argosy of professional viewpoints.

According to Dr. John Lukens, "The people he recruited were the best people I have ever worked with. I remember faculty meetings as being one of the high points of the week."[19]

The field of hematology/oncology may best exemplify the extraordinary changes occurring in medicine during that period. During the Christie era, very little could be done for children with such cancers as acute lymphocytic leukemia (ALL) and non-Hodgkins lymphoma. Surgeons could remove solid tumors in the operating room. Radiologists could mark up children with striking blue lines and then deliver a heavy dose of radiation in what was known as "cobalt bomb therapy." But chemotherapy was in its infancy as a treatment option, and Amos Christie and others considered it draconian.

John Lukens came to the Children's Hospital in 1975 as Vanderbilt's first nonsurgically trained hematologist/oncologist, and he had faith in the efficacy of chemotherapy. At that time, few children with leukemia were admitted to Vanderbilt Hospital because nearly all were referred to St. Jude Hospital in Memphis.

Many physicians couldn't fathom why Karzon would divert precious dollars to hire someone with Lukens's background. In fact, shortly after he arrived, Christie, by then an emeritus professor, attended a grand rounds Lukens was giving on new approaches to treating ALL. Christie challenged Lukens's assertion that leukemia was a curable disease and questioned the ethics of investing medical resources, hospital days, blood, and professional attention on such a small group of children.

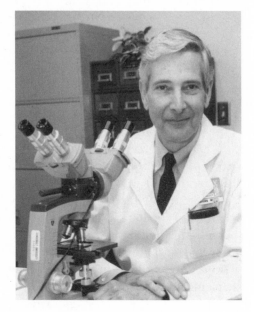

Dr. John Lukens.

"I learned shortly afterwards that he had never allowed a child with a malignancy to be transfused on his service," Lukens said. "He believed that they should be offered compassion and comfort, but their lives should not be prolonged."

Still, Christie was haunted by the data Lukens was presenting. He later came by the hematologist's office to talk. In his hand Christie held a graph which mapped the temperature curve of a child he had taken care of with ALL. The child had died with uncontrolled fever and severe anemia, and

Christie had always felt guilty that this had happened on his watch. Lukens looked at the graph and explained how he would have treated this same child.

"What you did was commendable for that time," Lukens told the senior physician, "but we can do more with this disease now."

From that point on, Christie began to trust that John Lukens indeed was on the path to not only treating but actually *curing* many children with leukemia. Lukens began working alongside Vanderbilt's surgical oncologists as well as town pediatricians in developing patient protocols for children diagnosed with cancer.

Lukens remarked:

> You treat a disease like a fatal disease and lo and behold it turns out to be fatal. You treat it with hope for a cure and more aggressively than you otherwise would, and lo and behold they are cured.
>
> It was one miracle after another. Suddenly these children with leukemia had been off treatment for five years and we began to call that a cure. And then the same thing began to happen with Hodgkin's Disease and non-Hodgkin's lymphomas, and a whole variety of metastatic germ cell tumors. Most of them were curable with chemotherapy alone.
>
> When I started off in oncology, the cure rate for children was about 20 percent. The cure rate at the time I retired was close to 80 percent. It has been remarkable to be part of the effort that made that possible.[20]

Tom Graham participated in similar advances in pediatric cardiology. In the early 1970s, physicians could only palliate or partially treat a high percentage of complex heart problems. Within twenty years, he said, they were able to treat virtually every child with a childhood heart disease.[21]

As the department evolved, money and the distribution of scholarly funds remained a thorn in the side of David Karzon. He insisted that physicians on his staff begin charging patients as they did in other parts of the country. The compensation schedule, however, proved to be unfairly biased. It worked to the benefit of certain clinicians and certain subspecialties, and to the detriment of researchers and those subspecialties based primarily on evaluation. Karzon knew that all of his faculty members were excellent physicians. He made an executive decision to redistribute departmental funds from the Vanderbilt Private Practice Plan so that both clinicians and research-oriented physicians were more equally compensated.[22]

The relationship between pediatrics and pharmaceutical companies was another aggravating issue. Amos Christie had tossed many a drug rep out of his office, determined not to sully the reputation of his department with money derived from sweetheart deals. Karzon, on the other hand, viewed relationships with drug companies as a necessary evil.

Beginning in the early 1970s, Bill Bell worked for Ross Pharmaceuticals, maker of Similac infant formula. He knew both Christie and Karzon—and he also knew the rules.

"The biggest difference between Christie and Karzon was that Karzon was a realist," Bell said. "Times had changed. Money had become a factor."

Karzon wanted his department and the Children's Hospital to grow, which was going to require dollars funneling in from a wide range of sources. He knew that sales reps were less interested in Vanderbilt's success than in gaining access to the residents, who would soon leave the institutional nest and embark into private practice. Karzon called Bell into his office and laid down the law. The pediatrician-in-chief told Bell:

> Fact of life: drug companies are here. Fact of life: your companies have a lot of money. Fact of life: you want access to my residents. Fact of life: I don't want you teaching my residents, because that's what I do. So we're going to play a ballgame that's about chasing dollars. I'm not going to shut you out, but I am going to tell you the rules of the game. I want you to stop wining and dining my people. You've got money to spend on them and I'm going to tell you how to spend it. There's no tit for tat, no quid pro quo. If you support pediatrics, I'll let you in the hospital and I'll let you talk on a scientific level with my residents. But I'll not tolerate you making a pitch to my residents about Similac.
>
> You're going to go in there and if my residents request that you give them Similac, that's between you and them. But we'll have rules and standards, and if you violate them, I'll kick you out of my hospital.

Given that the game plan had been clearly laid out from the start, Bill Bell and Vanderbilt pediatrics had a fruitful thirty-year relationship.[23]

As he delved into unknown waters, Karzon was keenly aware that he was being scrutinized by those skeptical of a major departmental overhaul. He knew he could not let slide the teaching and training component of pediatrics, which had become so solid under Amos Christie. While other institutions were rapidly hiring nurse practitioners (which was a relatively new field) to fill in the gaps in regional health care, Karzon chose to resist the trend and concentrate on his residency training. His idea was to build such a strong pediatric residency program that graduates would want to stay close by and set up their practices in Middle Tennessee.

"That way," he said, "we'll have concentric rings of Vanderbilt-trained pediatricians that go out from the Children's Hospital, and those physicians will give us a network of referrals."[24]

Much of the residency training took place at Nashville General Hospital. When Dr. Buck Donald stepped down as the solitary pediatrician-in-residence at Nashville General, Karzon received a call from a former Vanderbilt medical student and resident, William Altemeier, who was on faculty at the University of Florida. Altemeier wanted to apply for the job. Karzon had a unique interviewing technique. He would take the candidates to Centennial Park and they would sit by the lake in his car and talk about their dreams for their lives, their careers, and for the future of medicine.

Altemeier was sold. He took a pay cut and arrived at Nashville General as its only attending pediatrician, in charge of four interns and three residents, with whom he would run the entire service. Nashville General was almost strictly a charity hospital then, and the doctors who rotated through there essentially were on call twenty-four/seven.

"It was really fun," Altemeier remembered. "You saw something different every day. You had to watch everything that was going on and head off a crisis at any minute."

One such crisis occurred late one Friday night. He had already returned home and was getting ready to pop open a can of beer when he got a phone call from his resident, Dr. Jennifer Najjar.

"Have you ever sent the wrong baby home with the wrong mother?" Najjar asked him.

Altemeier answered that no, he'd never done that.

"Well," she said, "you have now."

"I'll be right there," Altemeier replied, putting down his beer.

It so happened that a frazzled nurse had accidentally placed the patient identification armband on the wrong child. Najjar realized that the name on the baby's armband didn't match the name on the bassinette. Regrettably, the baby in the bassinette had already been discharged. Altemeier called the police, who brought out a fingerprint expert to match the children's fingerprints, weight, and blood types.

"Yep," the expert announced, "they've been switched."

Altemeier went to the mother whose baby had been discharged, explained what had happened, and asked for the child in her arms. Assuring her that he would bring her rightful child back as soon as he could, the mother calmly handed over the infant. "I thought that baby looked a little different," she said.

Altemeier, a nurse, and the baby then climbed into a patrol car with a police escort and began the sixty-mile drive across two counties. They were to deliver one child and retrieve the other one, who was at a house in the back country with no telephone, sleeping next to a woman who was not his mother. At 3:00 a.m. they reached the Davidson County line and had to transfer to a police car from the next county. When they finally got to the home, the policeman pounded on the door and woke up the sleeping woman. Altemeier explained that she had the wrong baby and that the child he was carrying was actually hers.

The mother gladly made the trade. "I thought that baby didn't look like mine," she said.

The convoy returned to Nashville General Hospital, where Altemeier gave the waiting mom her baby. Everything seemed to have turned out fine, until six that same morning when Altemeier got a call from the head of the hospital—who had just read about the mix-up in the *Tennessean*. Because they'd had to change cars, the Davidson County police had radioed for their next escort to meet them at the county line, which meant it was broadcast over the dispatch system and therefore available to be picked up by all the area newspapers.

The episode became a featured news item across Tennessee. In fact, a few days later, Altemeier suffered even further for his fifteen minutes of fame. He wound up on the front page of the *National Enquirer* under the headline, "Babies Switched!" After a few more flare-ups from the aftermath, he said, the whole ordeal ended without incident.[25]

In spite of such exciting events, transmutations, research discoveries, and medical advances happening inside its walls, and despite the best efforts of fund-raisers and marketers to increase its visibility, the new Children's Hospital continued to suffer from an impregnable identity crisis. Other than the Palm Sunday Paper Sale, which the Friends now ran, Nashvillians generally remained clueless about the place.

Two extraordinary interventions, however, rescued the Children's Hospital from the haze of obscurity. The first was Watergate. The second was an awkward embrace by the burgeoning country music industry.

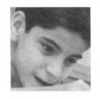

Establishing an Identity | 17

*"Country music artists are just like the rest of us.
They just keep different hours."*

**—Frances Preston, former head of the Nashville offices
of BMI, a publishing rights and licensing agency
for musicians and songwriters**

Tennessean editor John Seigenthaler tried his best to keep Vanderbilt's Children's Hospital in the spotlight. He sent his reporters off to write heartwarming stories about sick and recovering children. He published pieces about new doctors being hired and the strides being made in medical research. And he'd made sure that every year the *Tennessean's* part in the Palm Sunday Paper Sale went off without a hitch.

Still, he kept butting up against an ongoing problem that was giving him a full supply of headaches. Nearly every time that an article appeared in his newspaper, the phone on his desk started ringing. Either David Karzon, one of the ladies from the Junior League, or one of the Friends of Children's Hospital was on the line chewing him out because the reporter got the hospital's name wrong. Instead of the Children's Hospital at Vanderbilt, the story would read: "Vanderbilt Hospital," or worse, "Vanderbilt's pediatric unit."

Finally, Seigenthaler called his staff together and told them that either they were going to have to learn to separate the two hospitals or he was going to make them take all the irate phone calls. "Well, hell," a reporter told him after visiting what looked for all the world like a pediatric unit, "it *is* Vanderbilt Hospital!"

"No, it's *Children's Hospital!*" his editor sputtered. "It just looks like a pediatric unit!"

Seigenthaler also happened to live next door to Alice Ingram Hooker, a leader in both Friends and the Junior League. Sure enough, when a feature ran with the wrong name, Hooker would appear at his front door, frustrated and hopping mad. She had cause to be annoyed. This had been going on for nearly four years.

"Look, Alice, changing a culture is not easy," Seigenthaler told her.

Hooker said, "It's not just you, the *Banner* screws it up, television screws it up, too. Seig, you're supposed to be a smart guy. So, you tell us what can we do?"[1]

The truth was that at the moment Seigenthaler had bigger items on his plate. The aftershocks of Watergate were reverberating throughout the nation and Tennessee's senator Howard Baker was a major player. Although born and raised in a Democratic stronghold, Baker was Tennessee's first popularly elected Republican senator. During the Watergate hearings a few months earlier, he'd proved himself to be an intelligent, objective seeker of the truth, repeatedly asking the question, "What did the President know and when did he know it?"[2] Since he was handsome and charismatic, the media had termed him "the studliest senator in the Senate."[3] Baker was primed for higher office.

A brilliant idea flickered in Seigenthaler's brain.

He said:

> Alice, the way to get across that you have a hospital-within-a-hospital at Vanderbilt is to put the media on site. And the way to get the media there is to attract them on some hot subject. And the hot subject right now is Watergate, and the person they want to talk to is Howard Baker.
>
> Consequently, we have to get Howard Baker to come to the playroom of Children's Hospital, and we have to get it out there that Howard wants to talk about the Children's Hospital, and the importance of the name and the importance of the place.[4]

Seigenthaler knew that Baker was a good guy and would probably like the idea. The key was to invite the press to tag along while Baker toured the new Children's Hospital. He would give a short twenty-minute speech about how wonderful the place was, and then they would open up the press conference, no holds barred, to let members of the press pummel him with inquiries about Watergate and whether or not he was intending to make a run for the presidency.

"So," Seigenthaler concluded, "to solve the problem, you just need to call Howard Baker."

"Seig, I can't be the one to make that phone call," Hooker answered. "Howard knows I'm a Democrat!"

Fortunately, any number of women in the Junior League and Friends had a direct line to some of the most powerful Republicans in the state, and the phone call was made. Not only was he accommodating, recalled Alice Hooker, "Howard Baker was as game as Dick Tracy!"

On November 2, 1973, Baker appeared at Vanderbilt dressed in a dapper plaid jacket, his dark hair coiffed, and his long sideburns carefully styled. A throng of national and local journalists, photographers, and editors trailed his every move. Baker entered the Children's Hospital, which the Friends had festooned from top to bottom with paper doll cutouts. All the children were wearing buttons with the logo. The doctors had attached the buttons to their white coats, and Baker had a logo-laden nametag and button pinned upon

Senator Howard Baker conducted a health care tour to inform reporters about Vanderbilt's unique configuration of a children's hospital-within-a-hospital (left to right: Dr. John Chapman, Friends President Mary Henderson, Senator Howard Baker).

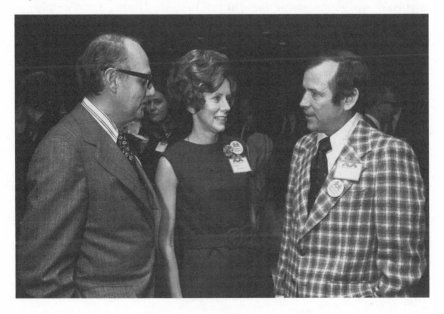

his lapel. The media lapped it up. Photographers' bulbs flashed, and given the high density of decorations, the children-holding-hands image showed up somewhere in every picture taken. The senator gave his speech, cheerfully answered their political questions, and posed for photos with hospitalized children along with Acting Dean John Chapman and Friends President Mary Henderson.[5]

The *Banner's* cutline proclaimed, "The unique arrangement of the medical unit provides the Children's Hospital as a hospital within a larger hospital to give broad health services to the young." The event was even given the weighty headline of Howard Baker's "Health Care Tour."

Seigenthaler recalled, "It worked! It finally impressed upon people that, yes, this is an identifiable wing, and it is a children's hospital and there's nobody in it except children."

Alice Hooker admitted, "It was an ingenious idea. People poured in there. It was a good deal for everybody."

Establishing an identity wasn't the only uphill battle that the Children's Hospital faced year after year. When the Friends organization first formed, one of its goals was to include all segments of the local population. They'd succeeded in embracing the upper-crust Protestant, the Jewish, and the African American populations, but never quite managed to interest the folks running the Nashville music industry. On an individual basis, certain artists had always been involved with patients at the Junior League Home, the Council of Jewish Women's Convalescent Home, and now at the Children's Hospital at Vanderbilt. Dinah Shore, Minnie Pearl, and Johnny Cash were among the regular visitors donating their time to entertain the children,[6] and Hank Snow approached David Karzon about setting up programs to prevent child abuse.[7] Also, music industry executives like Owen Bradley and Irving Waugh served on the Board of the Children's Hospital. Still, the Friends could never quite get a grip on the unwieldy talent residing only a few blocks away on Music Row.

The Belle Meade denizens, in particular, had issues with the rockabilly culture for which their town was known. Which is not to say they never capitalized on it. In 1962, the Junior League of Nashville hosted the regional conference for its members with the theme, "Framework for the Future." Party invitations, cut from felt in the round shape of 45-records, extolled the secondary theme of "Music City, U.S.A."[8] In truth, most high-society Nashvillians were apt to be as familiar with Patsy Cline as with Caruso and with songs written by

Harlan Howard as by Mozart. The main issue they had with country music in terms of fund-raising was that country stars tended to sing about lovin', lyin', cheatin', and drinkin'—and they were often basically living their lyrics. Of course, well-to-do people were having the same experiences—they just weren't looking for airplay.

The person who truly bridged the gap, beginning in the late 1960s, was Frances Preston, president of the Nashville office of Broadcast Music, Inc. (BMI). The mission wasn't easy, she said. For example, one year BMI brought the American Symphony Orchestra League to Nashville for a conference of symphony conductors from all across the United States. Preston had asked the conductors what kind of music they wanted to hear at the sponsored party, and they requested a performance by Chet Atkins. Although Atkins was best known for his country and bluegrass licks, he was also exalted for his brilliance as a classical guitarist. The party for the Orchestra League members was held at Cheekwood, the bluestone mansion-turned-museum, and was hosted by Walter Sharp, founder of the Nashville Symphony and whose wife was a descendant of the original family that had made its fortune by creating the Maxwell House coffee brand.

On the night of the event, Chet Atkins arrived at Cheekwood and was met by Walter Sharp, who was greeting people at the door. Sharp took one look at the humbly dressed Atkins and sent him around to enter by way of the kitchen.

"Chet was so upset," Frances Preston related. "I spent most of my night in the kitchen convincing Chet Atkins that it didn't matter what Walter Sharp said, the conductors of the nation's symphonies knew who he was and really did want to hear him play!"[9]

Because the Friends officers were juggling a virtual house of cards with the hospital-within-a-hospital, they felt they had to be extremely cautious in selecting the people who represented them. Sometimes they were a little too cautious. In 1974, the group wanted to tap into the opening of the new Grand Ole Opry House built on the grounds of Opryland by holding a concert benefiting the Children's Hospital. Dean Reeves was in charge of the show—a fun, lighthearted evening with Lawrence Welk serving as guest conductor with the Nashville Symphony Orchestra. Welk, who by that time had retired from television and his ubiquitous *Lawrence Welk Show*, brought along the clarinet and piano players from his band.[10]

"People are tired of hard music," he said in a preperformance interview.

As it turned out, they were not that tired. The Friends struggled to get people to buy tickets. Friends members went out and "begged and pleaded,"[11] but Lawrence Welk was not the draw they'd anticipated. "We got people to come, but it was scraping the bottom of the barrel," Carole Nelson admitted.

After their heroic efforts to sell tickets, Nelson was among those relieved to finally make her way to the concert. She felt beautiful. All the women were wearing long gowns and hers was a pale pink. As

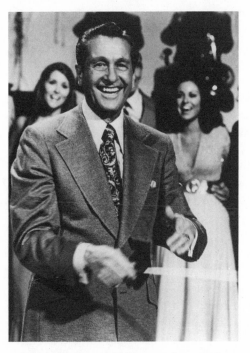

The Friends were hard-pressed to find a celebrity clean-cut enough to launch a fundraiser for Vanderbilt Children's Hospital until they signed Lawrence Welk to perform at the newly opened Grand Ole Opry House.

she was walking through the parking lot under the bright Opryland lights, a voice behind her called out sharply, "Carole!" She turned around to face an indignant Hortense Ingram.

"Carole, you did not wear a petticoat!" Ingram snapped.

"Mrs. Ingram, I did!" Nelson said apologetically, lifting up the hem of her dress to show her the petticoat underneath.

"Well, when you walk I can see straight through your dress!" Hortense Ingram told her. "I can see your legs!"

Needless to say, Nelson was horrified. She went in and sat down on the front row, afraid to move. During the performance, Welk decided to incorporate a bit of his familiar stage business into the show. He went into the audience and, seeing a lovely lady in pink on the front row, grabbed Carole Nelson by the hand and began to pull her up to dance with him on the stage.

"No, no," she hissed at him. "I can't go up there. You can see through my dress!"

Apparently, Welk had gotten either a little hard of hearing or a little mean in his later years because he ignored her. Up she went, waltzing with Lawrence Welk, her head bent down towards his shoulder so that nobody could see how she was blushing. All of those friends, neighbors, and colleagues, whom she'd worked so hard to put in their seats, gazed in disbelief as Carole Nelson danced under the glowing stage lights in her see-through dress.[12] Legend has it that this was the highlight of the evening.

The Friends used the $5,208 raised at the Lawrence Welk benefit concert to purchase fifty-seven recliner chairs for the pediatric rooms so that parents would have a place to sleep while their children were in the hospital.[13]

Several years later, even after country music was in a boom phase, the Friends still felt compelled to tread lightly when it came to protecting the image of the Children's Hospital at Vanderbilt. Ed Nelson was chairman of the Children's Hospital Board when he received a phone call from Irving Waugh, who headed up WSM Radio, the anchor station for the Grand Ole Opry. Waugh could hardly contain his enthusiasm. He had connections with Linda McCartney, wife of former Beatle Paul McCartney, who was interested in holding some benefit performances. During the 1970s, the Beatles had gone to India, experimented with certain mind-altering drugs, returned to the Western Hemisphere, and broken up as a band. McCartney had recently been busted for possession of marijuana and, said Waugh, as part of his penance was willing to come to Nashville, give a concert, and donate the proceeds to Vanderbilt Children's Hospital.

Ed Nelson was ecstatic. He called the Friends organization, where his wife was still an officer, and told them the news. Essentially, the response he got was, " um . . . thanks, but no thanks . . . we don't think Paul McCartney with his drug problems and his reputation would fit in with the image of the Children's Hospital."

Nelson said, "I was glad to get a quick answer, at least. But I had to tell Irving Waugh."[14]

"We could not, at that point, have a benefit by someone who openly enjoyed marijuana," explained Carole Nelson. "There was too much risk to it."[15]

Frances Preston finally got the two sides speaking something close to the same language when she, Helen Farmer, and Wesley Rose, who headed up Acuff-Rose music publishing house, suggested that the music industry people put on a three-day charity event during the weekend prior to the Country Music Awards show. They would sponsor golf, bowling, and tennis tournaments for various charities, and the proceeds from the tennis tournament would go to the Children's Hospital. The Friends and hospital board members jumped at the chance to become the beneficiaries of the Music City Tennis Invitational.

"Suddenly, I was spending my whole week cutting out of yellow paper little 'children holding hands' to string along the tennis courts," Frances Preston said.

The tournament was set up so that artists, celebrities, songwriters, and business people in the music industry would play against business people in the community at large. Immediately, 116 people signed up to participate, raising thousands of dollars in donations.[16] Perhaps more important, both groups got to know each other in a fun, semi-competitive environment. The local business community began to see the untapped revenues looming within the music industry and realized that they had been underestimating the business acumen of its leaders. In fact, the first real exchange of goodwill was initiated through area bankers, said Preston, "because they recognized that a lot of money was flowing through country music."

With that contact established, the Friends organization asked Preston to meet with them and advise them about ways to gain the attention of country music artists who might be willing to donate their time to charitable causes. Preston spoke to the Friends officers and minced no words.

"I had to explain that artists don't conform to organized giving," she said.

> They won't sit on the charity boards or attend all the meetings of the United Givers or the United Fund. They won't read all the literature and fill out all the forms. They will give of their talent and they'll turn loose of their money when they find something that really touches them. They often give because something arouses their passion, and they often give in ways that offer them no recognition. They're good people.

"Country music artists are just like the rest of us," Preston explained. "They just keep different hours."[17]

With the ground rules more clearly understood, the Friends and Vanderbilt Children's Hospital established a mutually respectful, invaluable relationship with the country music industry. Through the decades, that relationship has only grown stronger.

By the end of the 1970s, the Palm Sunday Paper Sale was beginning to lose some of its luster.[18] It still served as the primary fund-raiser for the Children's Hospital and drew in people from all walks of life; however, many of Nashville's bourgeoisie, who'd been actively involved during their salad days, were beginning to grow weary of the event. Around the same time, a subset of this same crowd, the horse people, or those who raised thoroughbreds on their large spreads south of town, were seeking a charity to become the beneficiary of the Iroquois Steeplechase.

In steeplechase racing, jockeys run their steeds around an oval track that includes jumps and obstacles. The sport originated in Britain among hunters, who, after a day of shooting quarry, raced their horses home or to a local landmark like a church by jumping over shrubs, water holes, and fences. The race was later refined into a spectator activity and was so elite it earned the title, "the sport of kings."

Country music celebrities, such as Minnie Pearl and Riders in the Sky, were part of a long tradition of country music artists who performed for hospitalized children in Middle Tennessee.

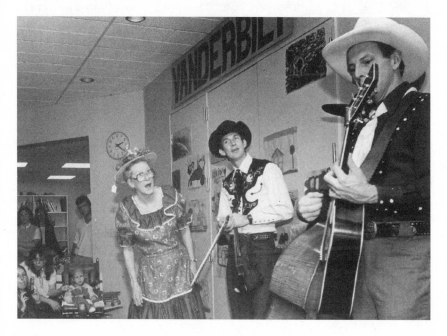

Steeplechase racing for purse money became a Nashville pastime in 1941. During the Depression, the government gave a controversial forty-five-thousand-dollar Works Progress Administration (WPA) grant to the city to build a steeplechase course (and later a twelve-thousand-dollar grant for a riding academy) at Percy Warner Park, the two-thousand-acre endpoint of the Belle Meade community. The donation was hardly the typical WPA contribution used to support needy families, financially strapped rural areas, and unemployed workers. In any case, the Iroquois Steeplechase quickly became a trendy annual event for the affluent in Nashville.[19]

By the mid-1970s, the second generation of race organizers was growing older just as the race itself was getting bigger, fancier, and more renowned. They were not only managing the event, but also managing the social functions surrounding it, such as the glamorous Hunt Ball, sparkling luncheons, and various glitzy parties held to appease the box holders who had come to town for the race.

"The horses were running for the money," said Alice Hooker, whose husband, Henry, was one of the major organizers. "The reason to charge for the boxes was always to get money to pay the purses."

While the organizers lost no interest in coordinating the race itself,

BMI Nashville President Frances Preston ran interference between the local music industry and the local business community by setting up fund-raising events like the Music City Tennis Tournament to benefit Vanderbilt Children's Hospital.

explained Hooker, "They were getting tired of having the parties. They wanted to control the event, but they wanted somebody else to do the work."

Since Alice Hooker had been actively involved in the Children's Hospital for years, she convinced the volunteers at Friends to take charge of the entertainment surrounding the Steeplechase. In return for sponsoring, planning, and hosting the associated luncheons and galas, the Children's Hospital would receive the money raised at the race. Vanderbilt administrators loved the idea of becoming connected with the Steeplechase's landed gentry and were thrilled to have so much visibility for the Children's Hospital. A more ticklish task, Hooker said, was convincing the horsemen to buy into the scheme.

"The horsemen were suspicious that Vanderbilt wanted to take over their event and be the boss," she said. "And to this day, the horsemen feel like they own the event and Vanderbilt is the invited guest."

Be that as it may, since its inception as a fund-raiser, the Iroquois Steeplechase has generated around $6 million in funds for Vanderbilt Children's Hospital. The purses for the riders now range from $10,000 to $150,000, depending on the race.[20] And the horses, which used to be traded for around seventy-five hundred dollars, are now each worth hundreds of thousands of dollars.

"The hardest job has been managing our success," Hooker remarked.[21]

By the late 1970s, the Children's Hospital at Vanderbilt had finally become what the Friends and Junior League had hoped it would become—an entity. Geographically, it was still spread all over the Medical Center, but the community rallied in support when fund-raisers were held via radiothons, telethons, and walkathons; through tennis tournaments, foot races, and horse races; and by sales of cards, Christmas tags, and Palm Sunday tabloids.

Yet, while the Children's Hospital was building its identity, the ladies of the Junior League were losing theirs. The greatest fears expressed by some of the sustaining members almost ten years earlier were starting to come true. True, the Junior League was still a pillar of the community. During the 1970s, the League became involved in programs with Family and Children's Services, the YWCA, and the Tennessee Environmental Council. Along with Nashville's Council of Jewish Women, the Junior League sponsored a statewide Bicentennial Arts Celebration. Also, the Home Unit at Vanderbilt always remained front and center. In fact, the League opened a brace shop adjacent to the physical therapy department in Vanderbilt Hospital.[22]

Still, without the Home for Crippled Children on White Avenue and without control of the Palm Sunday Paper Sale, the Junior League of Nashville seemed to be faintly ebbing away from the public consciousness.

That slow drift might have continued were it not for something that happened in 1977 that pushed the League to the brink of crisis. On that day, a local sheriff drove up to the organization's headquarters and served the group with a subpoena. Certain individuals were suing the Junior League of Nashville for money in its Trust Fund.

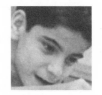

The Junior League of Nashville Stands Trial   18

*"Mary and Fran were such great witnesses that I
kind of felt sorry for the guys on the other side. Those
women were so charming. They had an answer for every
question. The other lawyers didn't stand a chance."*

**—Wilson "Woody" Sims,
attorney with Bass, Berry & Sims law firm**

Wilson "Woody" Sims had served as the counsel for the
Junior League for only a short while when he got his first
case. The League president called to inform him that the
Junior League of Nashville was being hit with its first lawsuit over
moving the Home for Crippled Children into Vanderbilt—even
though the merger had occurred years earlier. Sims, a founding
partner of the law firm Bass, Berry & Sims, was well entrenched in
Nashville. In fact, his wife was a member of the Junior League, so he
knew the principal players and the dynamic personalities. He immediately phoned Mary Stumb, who had been president of the League
during the crucial 1971–72 term. Sims asked her if she'd be willing to
testify. Of course, she answered, she'd be happy to.

Actually, Stumb and other members of the transition team had
been expecting this call for some time. Back when they were planning
to shift the physical residence of the Home to Vanderbilt, they had
established a steering committee to investigate all the legal ramifications and possibilities that might result from the decision. One of the
potential crises they anticipated was that someone might sue the
League for money in the Trust, claiming that the Home for Crippled
Children no longer existed.

"We got a lot of publicity in the paper about it moving from White Avenue to Vanderbilt Children's Hospital, and I'm sure [some people] at that point thought, 'Oh, good, maybe we can get this money,'" Stumb said. "So, no, we were not surprised. I was a little surprised we didn't have *more* [lawsuits]."

In the summer of 1970, the League's treasurer Fran Hardcastle was pregnant with her third child and had been put on complete bed rest due to early complications. Knowing she was captive, Stumb had gone over to Hardcastle's house with a box full of all the wills that went into the Trust and handed them over to her saying, "Here's something for you to do! Read these!"[1]

"I am the only human who has read all those wills to make sure that there were no red flags a layperson saw in what we were doing," Hardcastle said.[2]

Her job was to ensure that the League was using the money in the Trust not only according to the letter of the law, but also for the intent of the testator. If the bequest resulted in a surplus of funds, she made sure that the extra funds were appropriately allocated.

Woody Sims asked Fran Hardcastle to testify, too.

Prior to moving the Junior League Children's Home to Vanderbilt, the organization had settled fairly easily a number of legal challenges to the Trust. Most of those involved laypeople, who had left handwritten documents bequeathing, for example, their property and tools to the "crippled children's home of Nashville, Tennessee," or their estates to "the crippled children." If the deceased had donated to the Junior League Home for Crippled Children during their lifetimes, the court usually ruled that they meant for their estates be turned over to the Junior League of Nashville rather than to distant relatives.[3]

Having the Crippled Children's Home at Vanderbilt, however, presented a new set of challenges that would not be settled so easily. In July 1977, the Chancery Court of Cannon County, Tennessee, at Woodbury heard a case filed against every group that had ever had any relations with the Crippled Children's Home, including the national headquarters of the Imperial Council of the Shrine of North America, the Shriners Hospitals for Crippled Children, Vanderbilt University, and the Junior League of Nashville. Virginia A. Charter had died in 1976 with no surviving husband or children, leaving a paper purporting to be her last will and testament. Her next of kin argued that Mrs. Charter had left her assets to a nonexistent recipient, since her will stated, ". . . after all bequeaths [*sic*] have been made, the remainder of my estate be give [*sic*] to the shriners home for crippled children in Nashville, Tenn. [*sic*] . . ."[4] Because the Shriners had no such hospital in Tennessee, the heirs felt they deserved to inherit all of Mrs. Charter's property.

On the trial date, attorney Sims drove his witnesses down to the courthouse in Woodbury and put Fran Hardcastle and Mary Stumb on the stand to testify. "How would you like to cross-examine Mary Stumb or Fran Hardcastle when they knew ten times as much as you about a subject?" Sims asked rhetorically.

These two women knew the history and the operation of the Junior League Home inside and out. They responded to every inquiry with confident, cultured diplomacy. Not only did they own the facts, but according to their lawyer, they actually had a little fun on the witness stand.

Sims said, "Mary and Fran were such great witnesses that I kind of felt sorry for the guys on the other side. Those women were so charming. They had an answer for every question. The other lawyers didn't stand a chance."[5]

The judge instructed both sides not to discuss the case during the lunch recess. Whereupon, Sims, Hardcastle, Stumb, the plaintiffs' attorneys, and the judge all went across the street to a little restaurant on the square, sat at the same table, and ate lunch together.

"It was a friendly group," Hardcastle recalled. "Each one definitely wanted to win his own case, but we were aware it was not personal. Everybody was still pleasant."[6]

At the end of the day the judge ruled in favor of the Junior League. In his decree he wrote:

> The Court finds that the Home, the intended beneficiary, is presently existing, supported financially and otherwise by the Junior League, as part of the Vanderbilt Children's Hospital, where it is carrying on substantially the same services as it performed at the time Mrs. Charter made her will.[7]

With that ruling, the Junior Leaguers began to think that the matter of the transfer of the Crippled Children's home was closed. Not so. A year later, the association was served with another subpoena, and this one was more complicated than the last. In the 1950s, Davidson Country resident Goodloe Cockrill probated a will

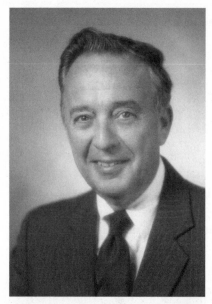

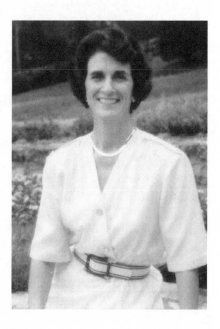

When people sued to obtain money in the Junior League Trust Fund, attorney Wilson "Woody" Sims (top) enlisted sustaining members Fran Hardcastle (below left) and Mary Stumb (below right) to serve as expert witnesses. Ultimately, the Supreme Court of Tennessee ruled in favor of the Junior League of Nashville.

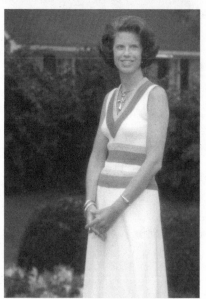

leaving fifty thousand dollars in a trust fund at a local bank from which his son, Sterling, could draw interest until his death. Upon Sterling's death, the will stated, the Cockrill Trust would continue for a period of twenty-five years and "therefrom shall be used for the benefit of the Junior League Home for Crippled Children in Nashville. . . ."[8]

By 1961, Goodloe Cockrill had added additional codicils to his will, including the caveats that if the Junior League of Nashville discontinued operation of the Crippled Children's Home, then "the Trust shall be null and void" and the fifty thousand dollars would go to Sterling; however, if Sterling had died in the interim, then the money would be distributed to Goodloe Cockrill's grandchildren. Goodloe died in 1964 and Sterling died in 1976, never having contested his father's will or having attempted to terminate the trust. Goodloe's grandchildren, on the other hand, were ready for combat.

In all likelihood, the ensuing legal scuffles stemmed from one disastrous conversation. The fable goes something like this: When it came time to execute Sterling's will upon his death, the bank holding the trust made a phone call to the Junior League headquarters. "Is there still a Crippled Children's Home on White Avenue?" asked the caller.

"No," came the response, "the children have moved to Vanderbilt."

The caller then phoned a department at Vanderbilt University. "Is the Junior League Home for Crippled Children over there?" the person asked.

"Nope. I've never heard of it," the Vanderbilt employee said.[9]

And in one fell swoop, the battle lines were drawn.

With the approval of attorneys for both sides, Special Chancellor Jim Dale heard the case in Nashville on February 14, 1978. In the courtroom, Mary Stumb and Fran Hardcastle leaned over and whispered to Woody Sims, "That guy's daughter Karin was a big officer in the Junior League!"

In fact, Judge Dale's daughter, Karin Dale Coble, had been the president of the Junior League for the 1973–74 term. Which might have tipped the scales, except that three of the trial lawyers, Ovid Collins, George Bishop, and Thomas Evans, had wives who were also members of the League—as did Woody Sims.

"It was sort of a family fight, so to speak," Sims said.

In truth, it would have been difficult to try any case in Nashville without somebody having at least one relative who belonged to the Junior League. The wives of Nashville's lawyers gravitated to the organization. So, the case proceeded.

Judge Dale posited that the primary question to be decided was: Does the Junior League of Nashville continue to operate a convalescent home for children? Sims argued that the main issue was actually whether Goodloe Cockrill, in writing his will, desired to benefit the crippled children in Tennessee.

"If his purpose was to serve crippled children, then even if the Junior League had gone plumb out of existence, the Court could probably pick another trustee to do this," Sims stated. He went on to submit that even if that weren't the case, the Junior League Home for Crippled Children was, in fact, still in existence and operating on D-3100 at Vanderbilt Children's Hospital.

Attorney Bishop argued that the Home ceased to exist as soon as it transferred to Vanderbilt University because Vanderbilt had taken over the responsibility of caring for those children. Therefore, the fifty-thousand-dollar corpus of the trust should go to the children of Sterling Cockrill.[10]

Sims called Mary Stumb to the witness stand. She explained upon questioning that the facility on White Avenue was no longer a convalescent home but was now being used for the RIP, or Regional Intervention Progress program, and that the Dede Wallace Center for Mental Health was also located on that property. Stumb answered that yes, she had been actively involved in the Junior League and had served as president from June of '71 until June of '72. The testimony continued:

> Sims: And are you still active in the Junior League and its programs?
> Stumb: The Junior League of Nashville has a policy when a young lady reaches forty years of age, she becomes what is called a sustaining member.
> Sims: I can tell already I asked the wrong question.
> Stumb: I am still active in my participation, but I'm not classified as active. That's an unfair question, Mr. Sims.
> Judge Dale: She looks like she's still eligible![11]

Under questioning, Stumb continued to detail the history of the local organization, the scope of its reach across forty-one counties in Middle Tennessee, and the reasons for the merger with Vanderbilt Children's Hospital. She explained that prior to the transfer, Vanderbilt had no children's convalescent center and the majority of the staff from the Home was now working on the Junior League Home Unit at Vanderbilt Children's Hospital. All the activities, from recreation therapy to nursing to tutorial assistance that had been offered at the Home were now offered at the Home Unit. In addition, the Junior League was underwriting the entire salary of one physical therapist, one recreational therapist, and part of the salary for two social workers. The League was also paying for the convalescent care for indigent and uninsured children admitted to the ward. Since the merger agreement in 1970, Stumb informed the court, the Junior League had donated around $1 million to the operation of the Home Unit at Vanderbilt. In addition, thirteen of forty members of the Children's Hospital Board were also Junior League members, she said.

Sims handed her a list of Children's Hospital board members with checkmarks by the names of men whose wives belonged to the League. He quipped, "But I'm sure that the Junior League members have no influence on the decisions of their husbands."

Stumb coyly replied, "I would not like to answer that."[12]

The plaintiffs' attorneys then cross-examined Stumb, pointing out that Vanderbilt owned the physical facility where the Home Unit was housed, Vanderbilt cut the checks to pay the salaries of the Home Unit employees, and Vanderbilt handled all the third-party payments for the patients. Attorney Bishop asked the witness why in 1970 the Junior League had amended the contract for the original trust, striking out the clause that the trust would be terminated . . . "[i]n the event the Junior League of Nashville, Inc. shall for any reason whatsoever cease to own and operate said Home for crippled children. . . ."[13]

Stumb responded:

> . . . There were two reasons. One, we wished to move the Home to a facility that we no longer owned, and we wished to keep the Trust intact where the income from it still would go to these children, even though we didn't own the property in which the Home was to reside. The second reason for changing the Trust was that the White Avenue property, which we did still own . . . was indeed to house children who had what in a polite sense could be termed behavioral or developmental problems. And we wanted to be sure that legally we were able to do both of those things. We had no intention, as you can see, because we haven't done so in the last seven years, of the income not continuing to go to the Home. It has.[14]

To the plaintiffs' attorneys, the critical word in the original contract was "said" Home, meaning the trust funds were valid only if they were used for those patients residing in the building on White

Avenue. Stumb countered that the contract was amended so that the White Avenue building would continue to be used for a civic purpose, namely to house emotionally disturbed children, but also so that the trust income would still be dedicated to children convalescing from crippling diseases, as it always had been.

On March 10, 1978, Judge Dale ruled in favor of the Junior League. Members of the League were elated—but not for long because the Cockrill family filed an appeal. On June 29, 1979, Judge Samuel Lewis heard the case in the Court of Appeals and reversed Chancellor Dale's decision (with concurrence by appellate Judges Henry Todd and Thomas Shriver, whose daughter-in-law Bertie Shriver just so happened to be an officer in the Junior League), citing the following:

> The record shows that . . . some of these [Junior League Trust] funds are used for purposes other than as directed by Goodloe Cockrill.
> Simply to call a unit of the Children's Hospital the Junior League Convalescent Home does not satisfy the terms of the Cockrill Trust.
> . . . The facts at bar are clear. The Junior League ceased to operate a home or hospital for crippled children in Davidson County during the life of Sterling B. Cockrill.[15]

The League ladies were devastated. For one thing, failing to win the appeals case meant that every dime in the Junior League Trust was suddenly in danger of being seized by some long-lost relative. But also, the women of the Junior League simply weren't used to losing.

Fortunately for them, the debate was not yet over. Woody Sims took the case to the Supreme Court of Tennessee and asked the highest court in the state to determine, first, whether the Junior League had used Goodloe Cockrill's Trust as he had intended, and second, whether the Junior League Home for Crippled Children continued to exist and operate. This supreme court's decision on these two questions, both sides knew, would mark the end of the line.

In his written decision, Justice T. Mack Blackburn stated that, in his will, Goodloe Cockrill did not appear to the Chancellors to be intending "to establish the trust for the *maintenance or operation*[16] of a home or hospital for crippled children." Rather his will implied that he wanted to give the Junior League an interest in the trust, so long as they operated a home or hospital to benefit the crippled children of the region. He cited Mary Stumb's statement that the League even amended the wording of the Trust contract so that the organization could continue to channel the income precisely to the children Goodloe Cockrill was interested in helping.

On April 7, 1980, Chancellor Blackburn of the Supreme Court of Tennessee found that ". . . the Junior League Children's Home had not been discontinued," reversing the Court of Appeals and sustaining the decision of the original trial court. As a result, the Junior League of Nashville was allowed to continue receiving the net income from Goodloe Cockrill's Trust for the use and benefit of the Home Unit, "as now conducted under said contract with the Children's Regional Medical Center."[17]

At last, the decision by the Supreme Court of Tennessee validated that the Junior League Home still existed in the form of a wing of the Children's Hospital at Vanderbilt.

"When we won the appeal, I guess I was not surprised, but I was very glad, because I thought it set a precedent," Mary Stumb said. "I thought, 'Good. I'm so glad we've won this case, because maybe it will discourage other people from trying to get money that should go to the children.'"[18]

To protect itself from further legal issues, and to more closely regulate funds paid into the Children's Hospital from the Junior League, the group reinstated the Home Board. Frances Jackson, who had been president of the League ten years earlier when merger negotiations began in earnest, was the first chair of the reinstalled Home Board. Jackson's return to a major office brought continuity to the League, which was opening up its membership by then and expanding in size.

Even more important, perhaps, the reinstatement of the Home Board also signaled the Junior League's return to prominence among the general public, Fran Hardcastle said. As long as the community could associate the League with its good works at the Home—which had continued during its ten-year residence at Vanderbilt Children's Hospital, but without much fanfare—people would not only donate to benefit the children on the unit but also to other worthy causes the League sponsored.

Hardcastle concluded, "The Home was a unifying, connecting element."[19]

By decree of the Supreme Court of Tennessee, the Junior League Home for Crippled Children was finally once again real—even as it operated as a wing within Vanderbilt Hospital. Also, by association, the ruling served as a legal endorsement of the scattershot Children's Hospital-within-a-hospital. David Karzon, Nelson Andrews, the Junior

League, the Friends, and all the others who had strategized, schemed, and reconnoitered could no longer be accused of hiding behind smoke and mirrors. After all, the Supreme Court of Tennessee had declared in its final ruling that Vanderbilt Children's Hospital was indeed an entity.

If people were truly going to recognize it as an independent hospital-within-a-hospital, however, it would need to be built from the ground up as such, rather than simply as an afterthought inserted into an existing structure. This would entail constructing a brand new building for the main hospital and carefully designing the Children's Hospital to reside within it. The type of person capable of undertaking that formidable task would have to be someone brash, confident, and unfazed by dissension, someone who already knew how to build a hospital, and someone who didn't mind stepping on a few toes to get it done—someone like Dr. Vernon Wilson.

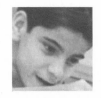

New Battles and Beginnings | 19

*"Vernon Wilson . . . came to Vanderbilt to build
a new hospital, come hell or high water. He did build
that hospital, and—you could ask anyone who was
around then—there was a lot of hell and high water."*

**—Jane Tugurian, executive assistant to
Vice Chancellor of Medical Affairs Dr. Vernon Wilson,
during his tenure at Vanderbilt**

Throughout its early, wobbly-legged years, saviors of Vanderbilt Children's Hospital emerged from a wide array of characters. At any given moment, the gauntlet might be taken up by a righteously indignant young mother dressed to the nines or by a grieving family member responding to personal tragedy. Sometimes rescuers assumed the form of driven academic physicians who refused to give up in the face of all obstacles. Or they appeared in the guise of concerned citizens, propelled, quite simply, by the belief that fighting for a children's hospital was a just cause for their community.

The strangest savior of all, however, might have been Dr. Vernon Wilson. When Wilson took over the office of vice chancellor of medical affairs in 1974, he soon made it known that he wasn't crazy about pediatrics as a specialty, he had issues with David Karzon and members of his staff, and he felt that, given all the crushing duties of his new job, the Children's Hospital deserved back-burner status. Ironically, in spite of these feelings, Wilson essentially saved the fledgling institution. At the very least, he cemented its entity as an integral yet independent hospital within the medical complex.

Although other leaders came from humble beginnings, Wilson was the only Teamster to ever head up Vanderbilt University Medical Center. Born and raised in an agrarian stretch of rural Iowa, Wilson skipped college during the Great Depression to help salvage the family farm by driving and repairing trucks for a printing plant. He joined the navy when World War II broke out, and after his tour, used his G.I. bill to enroll at a junior college in Minnesota at the ripe age of thirty-one. In 1951, he graduated with a bachelor's degree from the University of Illinois,[1] and then continued on a path that would define his preferred approach to any problem—by working from "four in the morning until ten at night." Using that formula, he earned both a master's degree in pharmacology and a medical degree in a record-setting span of two years.[2]

From there he held increasingly prestigious posts at the University of Kansas and the University of Missouri medical schools. Wilson's bailiwick was primary care medicine. He helped establish the Missouri Regional Medical Program for delivering top-flight medical care and information to stroke, cancer, and heart disease patients who lived in remote areas of the country removed from any major medical center. As early as the 1960s, Wilson had been studying how computers might be used in doctors' offices as tools for assisting in the delivery of health care.[3] In the early 1970s, he formulated national health policies as head of the Health Services and Mental Health Administration under Eliot Richardson. Such a job, chock-full of regulations and directives, suited his style.

In short, Wilson was a Midwesterner to the core—scrappy, Spartan, no-nonsense, impatient, and vastly productive. While he was not particularly imaginative, he was farsighted in a pragmatic and goal-oriented sense.

By 1973, the Vanderbilt administration recognized that Randy Batson, beloved as he may have been by the established faculty, was never going to plow through the maelstrom of decisions required of his position. The Board moved him into a role in development, named John Chapman as acting dean of the medical school, and launched a search for someone tough enough to move a cumbersome hierarchy by sheer force of personality.

Chancellor Alexander Heard was aware that the Medical Center was on the brink of collapse in a competitive marketplace that now included not only other Southern academic centers but a fertile chain of for-profit hospitals as well. The Vanderbilt facility, built in 1925, was in such poor condition that department chairmen couldn't attract the best candidates, the equipment and laboratory space were shamefully outdated, and nonindigent patients were choosing other options for health care services. Heard began patrolling for a medical vice chancellor unafraid to dish out some tough love. Fifty-nine-year-old Vernon Wilson was the embodiment of that ideal.

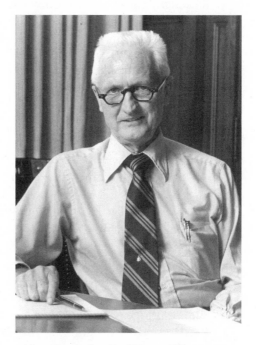

"Vernon Wilson . . . came to Vanderbilt to build a new hospital, come hell or high water," said Jane Tugurian, who was Wilson's executive assistant. "He did build that hospital, and—you could ask anyone who was around then—there was a lot of hell and high water."[4]

The Chancellor and the Board of Trust hired Wilson with the understanding that his mission was to figure out a way to finance and oversee the construction of not only a hospital but also a medical education building. The funding for the medical

Vice Chancellor Dr. Vernon Wilson came to Vanderbilt with one major goal—to build a new hospital on budget and within three years.

education building, finessed by Randy Batson, came as a gift from Vanderbilt alumnus Dr. Rudolph A. Light. The funding for the hospital, on the other hand, would require floating a few bonds.

Said James O'Neill, "Vernon Wilson had a proven track record in that regard. He knew how to build a hospital, how to get it funded, how to float bonds. Nobody here knew how to borrow money."[5]

Wilson's approach alarmed many people. In the 1970s, the total Vanderbilt endowment was $160 million. Wilson floated bonds against the endowment to pay the $52 million construction costs of the hospital—tying up over a third of the university's total capital. Many at Vanderbilt were sure that the hospital would never be able to recoup that investment, and they believed that after a full century of a rich and storied existence, Vanderbilt University was destined to go under.

That might have been the university's fate had not Wilson been so fixated on the task set before him. "Vernon was ruthless," O'Neill said.

> He was going to get that job done and if people got in his way, he fired them. Or he marginalized them. If you disagreed with him, if you didn't interact with him intellectually and forthrightly or if he didn't like you and didn't feel like you were dealing straight up, he'd develop an attitude and never change it.[6]

Wilson had little patience for politics or diplomacy. He didn't throw receptions for retiring physicians or roll out the welcome mat for new hires. In addition to a home in town, he and his wife, Ula, purchased a plot of land with a farmhouse out in the country, a tractor, and a backhoe. Every morning Wilson drove into work thinking about the new hospital. Every evening he returned home, thinking about the new hospital. On the weekends and in the long summer evenings, he'd head to his farm in Culleoka, Tennessee, and tour his spread on his tractor. If he had a particularly difficult problem to figure out, he'd spend hours immersed in the hard physical labor of baling hay—all the while thinking about the new hospital.[7]

The Board of Trust knew that the old hospital would hold up only for so long before Vanderbilt began losing medical students and embarking on a steady decline in research grants and patient loads. The board asked Wilson if, once ground was broken, he could get a large portion of the hospital built within five years. Wilson answered that he'd have the whole thing completed—on budget—in three.[8]

Invited to a luncheon given in his honor by Palm Sunday Paper Sale chairs Ann Miller and Frank Woods, Wilson sat through his introduction to the town's elite. Miller began, "You've all heard about our new Children's Hospital that's being built with completion to be in the 1980s . . ."

"I said *1980*," Wilson interrupted.

Miller continued, good-naturedly, ". . . [To] prove he's serious about it, he's bought a backhoe and he might just build the hospital himself."[9]

With many of the details still being hotly debated, the shovels hit the dirt in the summer of 1977 and construction commenced on the new university hospital. Twenty days later, Wilson suffered a heart attack and underwent cardiac bypass surgery. Two weeks after that, he was back on the job, as spry and as single-minded as ever.

Placed into the measured, erudite culture of Vanderbilt, Wilson was like a burr under the saddle of the research establishment. Doctors such as Mildred Stahlman, Grant Liddle, Bill Scott, and David Karzon were giants in their fields of medical research. Wilson was definitely not an academic physician, nor was he a researcher. What he recognized, said his former assistant Lewis Lavine, was that Vanderbilt had long placed so much emphasis on research and teaching that patient care was suffering—and after years of setting policy, he understood patient care upside down and sideways.

"You had an Old South cultured men's club at Vanderbilt, which was both good and bad," Lavine said.

> They were brilliant in their fields, they did great research, and they were incredible teachers. Patient care was not high on their list. Wilson was like a fish out of water—and he was at a point in his career where he didn't care. In fact, he seemed to enjoy jousting with the docs.[10]

According to Lavine, those doctors remained disconcerted most of the time Wilson was in office. If he had wanted to win friends, the vice chancellor's greatest tactical error was that he didn't put enough weight into the fact that he was an outsider. He rushed into his job focused on a goal without first getting a lay of the land. For example, he held numerous meetings with faculty members to discuss where to put the new hospital. Should it be on the same side of Garland Avenue as the old hospital, where there was very little available land? Or should they tear down the old hospital and put the new one in its place? Then again, they might put the whole building across the street where there was more room. He agitated and agonized over the decision. The faculty campaigned to build the new hospital on the same side as the existing Medical Center, in order to protect the unique aura of collegiality and intellectual exchange among the biomedical researchers, clinicians, and academicians so brilliantly fostered at Vanderbilt. Wilson, however, foresaw a modern era of medicine approaching. If Vanderbilt had the good fortune to make it under the wire, the Medical Center would be joining a fast-moving current and would need to expand.

"He had been in government long enough to understand national medicine and trends," Lavine said, "and he wanted to start Vanderbilt on a track to being a part of big-time medicine."[11]

Wilson turned autocrat and announced he was moving the new hospital across the street.

Having made that decision, he caused another uproar when he began contemplating out loud what to do with the Round Wing building. When David Karzon joined the Vanderbilt faculty, he had always intended to create a stand-alone children's hospital in town. After he settled for his hospital-within-a-hospital, knowing it was initially a marketing ploy to gain community support—which he had successfully done by the time of Wilson's arrival—he fully expected to be given the go-ahead to convert the Round Wing into a children's hospital, as promised, once the new hospital was up and running. That was not to be.

The new Vanderbilt University Hospital was designed to be in the shape of twin towers that would allow for future expansion.

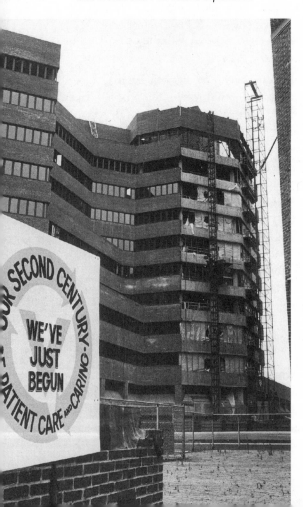

Although pediatrics occupied the third floor of the building, the cost of transforming the entire structure into a full-fledged free-standing children's hospital was astronomical. Wilson was already floating $52 million in bonds against the university's endowment. He was not going to embark on building two hospitals. Karzon was stunned—and profoundly dejected. To make matters worse, Wilson began testing the community waters to see if he could make the Round Wing building, as well as the D-Wing building connecting it to the Medical Center, available to the city. A task force convened to discuss whether the old Metro General Hospital might occupy that prime space.

Blithely unaware of the implications among the internal Vanderbilt faculty,

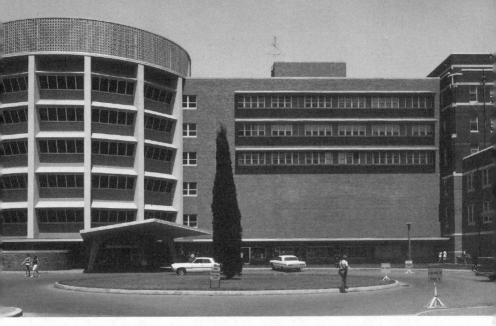

With the new hospital nearing completion, the Round Wing and D-Wing buildings suddenly came up for grabs as negotiable property.

Wilson told reporters that "the city—or at least the little-known health and hospital facilities board of Metro—holds title to the Round Wing already through the bonding agreements which built it."

He added that city officials foresaw a facility paid for by the city and run by the city "with Vanderbilt administrators 'staying across the street.'"[12]

Nelson Andrews had discovered a few years earlier that real estate to Vanderbilt personnel was the equivalent of sacred ground, and they had a habit of pouncing on anyone who threatened to take away—or even share—their space. Wilson was roundly condemned over his plans for the Round Wing, which ultimately stayed within the Vanderbilt domain. In 1983, several floors were converted into a pilot project burn center and rehabilitation facility.[13]

Wilson's willingness to option off the Round Wing, and by implication his pointed dismissal of the Children's Hospital, created a permanent rift with David Karzon. In all honesty, the two men were never going to get along. Karzon spoke slowly, fastidiously considering each word, and, as one of his faculty members described it, "took everything to the fourth decimal point."[14] Wilson had no time for belabored deliberations. He was in a hurry. He had a hospital to build. He tended to snap back at Karzon, who was used to being addressed with respect.

Wilson's raw-boned sense of humor also didn't sit well with Karzon. For example, Wilson believed that surgeons were not good at administrative details. The best way to keep surgeons happy, Wilson used to say, was to just "let 'em keep cuttin'."[15] Such humor was unnecessarily pejorative in Karzon's book.

The biggest differences between the two men, however, were philosophical. Since he'd arrived in Nashville, Karzon had been gaining disciples as he chanted the mantra, "Children are not little adults, and should not be treated as such." Wilson's career had been built upon primary care, where a single physician cared for a patient from birth through old age. Pediatric subspecialties, in his opinion, were going a little overboard in the art of medicine. Vanderbilt didn't have a primary care division in those days and Wilson thought that the Medical Center needed one. Karzon viewed it as stealing the thunder from pediatrics.

In the midst of their argument, Karzon suffered a back injury that left him in excruciating pain. For the better part of a year, he rarely came in to work for a full day, delegating from home instead and having his faculty members meet with him there.

Recalled Bill Altemeier:

> He had a swimming pool and in the spring he'd hold court and you'd come out there and sit on a chair and talk to him about things while he was lying on a picnic table beside his pool. It was the only position where he could get comfortable with his back pain.
>
> He was a very efficient meeting person. He was quick to understand the problem and quick to guide you through the decision-making process. These meetings were so informative that you were damn glad to have them. He got through the summer that way. Fall started to come. I was out there talking to him and leaves were falling all around. As the weather got colder, he'd still hold meetings on top of the table with a blanket on him. One time it started snowing, and, I swear, he was conducting business lying on his back with snowflakes falling on his face. I learned more from David Karzon than anybody except my father.[16]

Vernon Wilson had neither the time nor the sympathy for malingerers. Finally, he confronted the pediatric chairman and told him that he'd been absent for too many days and would have to choose between running his department or retiring from medicine in order to nurse his back. Not one for ceremony, Wilson then presented Karzon with data on how many days he'd been absent. The vice chancellor had been monitoring Karzon's attendance all along. Enraged, Karzon fought through the pain and returned to work. Wilson considered that appropriate, since, after all, he'd come back to his job within weeks of having cardiac bypass surgery.

In fact, David Karzon had had a rough go of it ever since Wilson was hired. Karzon's wife, Allaire, had left the small local law firm of Neal, Karzon, and Harwell to work as vice president and general counsel for Aladdin Industries under CEO Vic Johnson, a fellow Yale alumnus. While there, she received a phone call from the executives at her old company, RCA, in New York City. They asked her to move to New York and serve as a top attorney on their legal team. The offer was too glorious to refuse, so Allaire accepted the job, working and living in New York throughout the week and flying home to Nashville every weekend. By the end of two years of a commuter marriage, she was exhausted. In 1977, she called the dean of the Law School at Vanderbilt and told him she was thinking about returning to Nashville full-time and, if he had any openings, she would be interested in teaching tax law. Fortuitously, the dean was in the process of forming a search committee to find someone to teach that very subject. Allaire Karzon got the position and became Vanderbilt Law School's first full-time female professor.[17]

Over time, David Karzon's back injury began to heal, but the acrimony between him and Wilson never stopped percolating. Karzon, however, showed remarkable agility when confronted with bad news. Since the freestanding building was out of the question, he entered a pitched battle for everything he could get for the Vanderbilt Children's Hospital that was to be located on the fifth and sixth floors of the new university hospital.

To meet a limited budget, Wilson was cutting whatever corners he could. He gathered more data and discovered that the bed census at the Children's Hospital was erratic. Sometimes the beds were full and sometimes there were available beds, while the adult services were consistently bursting at the seams. Also, the highest percentage of bad debt write-offs was related to pediatric patients. The Pediatric and Neonatal Intensive Care Units, in particular, were found to be causing substantial losses to the hospital, which explained why other area hospitals were delighted to have Vanderbilt Children's Hospital carry that patient load.[18]

"Every time I see that Angel [neonatal transport van] come in," commented one of Wilson's financial advisors, "all I think about is the ten thousand dollars or fifty thousand dollars that Vanderbilt is losing."[19]

Wilson's solution was to reallocate certain pediatric beds to be used for adults when the demand arose. O'Neill stepped in as an intermediary, explaining that pediatric services were doing their best to keep those beds full and were achieving that goal as Karzon was hiring new subspecialists. Also, the department needed a full bed census, or a critical mass of patients, for pediatrics to meet its teaching obligations. He argued that chipping away at that critical mass would be detrimental to the educational effort.[20]

"I wrote that letter because I agreed with David that all of us who treated young patients would be stifled if the administration used pediatrics as a pop-off valve every time somebody needed a bed," O'Neill explained.

Despite the friction, O'Neill found Wilson surprisingly open-minded and reasonable during their debate. Eventually, Wilson agreed that pediatrics would not be able to expand and incoming subspecialists would not be able to admit to the service unless the bed census remained protected.

"I appreciated that attitude," O'Neill said. "So I hustled back to David and said, 'You gotta hurry up and recruit those physicians!'"[21]

In his quest to maintain control over his domain, Karzon maneuvered to have members of Friends of Children's Hospital appointed to the planning board. The whole concept of the Friends Board rubbed Wilson the wrong way. Karzon would meet with him, asking for more equipment, space, facilities, or resources for the Children's Hospital and Wilson would retort, "Go get it from the Friends."

Fran Hardcastle was on the planning committee of the board and emphasized that the Friends and the Junior League were behind the push to include a child-friendly quality to the design of the Children's Hospital. "We were still fighting for sleeper chairs and telephones in the rooms and the amenities that address family-centered care," she recalled. "The head doctor would call and say, 'There's going to be a meeting at four today.' I had three children and that was the worst time of day for me, but come hell or high water, I was going to be there. You knew they didn't want us to come."[22]

Carole Nelson also was a member of that committee, representing the interests of the Friends. Nelson had a personal stake in getting involved in the building design. It was a matter of gratitude. Vanderbilt doctors had saved the lives of her children.

In 1966, Nelson, her husband, Ed, and their daughters, five-year-old Carole and two-year-old Emme, were driving down Harding Road when a large cement truck came barreling down a hilly side street, out of control, and sideswiped the family station wagon. Carole

Nelson was thrown from the car and knocked unconscious. The younger Carole had asphalt burns and a head injury. And little Emme lay under the wheel of the truck, her skull shattered, her left leg torn halfway off, and her shoulder broken. An ambulance rushed them to Vanderbilt Hospital. Once they left the emergency room, the staff placed them together in the birth defect area of the Round Wing, where they had a room that could accommodate all three people with such severe injuries. Emme, whose injuries were the most traumatic, underwent hours of surgery to repair her fractured skull and to set her broken leg and shoulder. The family lived in the Vanderbilt Round Wing for months as, one by one, they recovered. Dr. William Meacham, Emme's neurosurgeon, said, "Every doctor has a miracle or two, and Emme Nelson is one. . . ."

In the end, both children survived without any major long-term damage other than the scars left from their wounds.[23] Having lived through that nightmare, Carole Nelson felt she owed it to the doctors at Vanderbilt and to the parents of injured children to advocate for them as the plans for the Children's Hospital began to roll out. For a year and a half, she attended the meetings without opening her mouth, mostly because the virile discussions centered around labyrinthine blueprints and architectural plans and installation features that had become obsolete before the first brick was laid. One day, she finally raised her hand.

"There's something that bothers me," she told the committee. "Why does the door to the patient's room open this way?"

One of the architects curtly explained that the way they had it designed was the most efficient way for the door to open.

"But," she persisted, "if you open the door the other way, the child is never out of the line of vision of the health care worker or the parent. If you open it the way it is here, the baby is behind the door."

Carole Nelson knew what it was like to stand behind that door, looking in at a critically wounded child. Each day for months she had taken a moment to brace herself for what she was about to see when she went into her daughter's room. Every parent, she insisted, deserved that one small favor. The architects relented and changed all the doors. And Carole Nelson felt like she had finally made a contribution to the design of the new hospital.[24]

Vernon Wilson liked to tell people that his leadership style was to "manage by exception," meaning, leave alone those things that are working and focus on those things where one can personally make a difference. For many years, the rule setters at Vanderbilt

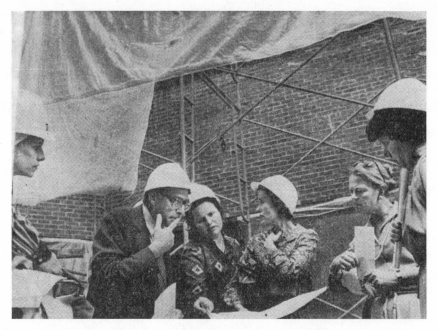

The Friends of Children's Hospital insisted on helping to design the new pediatric hospital-within-a-hospital and outdoor play area (left to right: Mrs. Edward Nelson, Dr. David Karzon, Mrs. Henry Hooker, Mrs. Ridley Wills II, Mrs. John McDougall, and Mrs. Eugene Swallow Jr.). Photo by Jimmy Ellis, Tennessean, *April 5, 1979.*

had considered Millie Stahlman's acclaimed sheep experiments to be off-limits. Wilson, however, put a stop to the long tradition of allowing her sheep to graze in the hospital courtyard. He suffered her wrath for that edict, but he stood by his decision.[25]

Despite his claims of ruling by exception, when it came to the new hospital, Wilson was the consummate micromanager, fretting over and demanding to sign off on the minutest details—the color of the drapes, the types and configurations of the beds, the wall colors and decorative murals. Meanwhile, the Friends Board had formed a subgroup called the New Hospital Liaison Committee to lobby for the needs and interests of the 125-bed Children's Hospital. After years of being involved with the Junior League Home and the original hospital-within-a-hospital, its members were experts in micro-management, and they proceeded as they had in the past—which is, they assumed they had infinite power until someone told them other-wise. The Liaison Committee campaigned for separate entrances into the main hospital lobby, separate elevators up to the fifth and sixth floors of the Children's Hospital, different decor for the registration and waiting area near the admitting office, specific furnishings for the surgical ward (including a mobile workbench), desks for the children to use for studying, and a storage unit in each room for toys.[26]

Immediately, the designers and architects began scrambling to meet the demands of the Liaison Committee, until Vernon Wilson fired off a memo saying that no action should be taken based on the committee's review. "The Hospital Liaison Committee functions as an advisory group to the Management Committee," Wilson asserted. "It is not an independent planning group, nor can it possibly be."[27]

The Liaison Committee was later shown a mock-up of a typical room in the Children's Hospital, garnering this response from Alice Hooker, chair of the Children's Hospital Board:

> . . . The shelf and cabinet space for the patient's possessions, flowers, toys or what have you is totally inadequate . . . The wall mural is attractive but not particularly appropriate . . . The bathroom is a disaster . . . It is an awkward and unattractive design as laid out . . . The Liaison Committee would hope that the many clever professionals responsible for this room design can significantly improve its present status.[28]

The Children's Hospital Board continued to jockey with Wilson for power when he demanded to have oversight of the fifth floor outdoor play area. In a gracious act of goodwill, the Wills family chose to donate funds to build a small playground in honor of their deceased son Jesse. Still, the vice chancellor wanted final say over the color and type of paving stones, the size and shape of the box planters, the lighting, the commemorative sculpture, and the playground activity equipment. Reams of paperwork passed among Wilson, the landscape designers, the volunteer playground design committee, and the Wills family before he signed off on the playground.

Despite all the spats that arose because of his rough-and-tumble style, Wilson slowly gained the admiration of many of the city's leaders. He had a salt-of-the-earth aura about him that gradually drew in a cadre of devotees. One of Wilson's first breakthroughs in that direction occurred when he approached Nelson Andrews and asked why Vanderbilt didn't have a donor society. After all, Vanderbilt was building a new hospital to serve patients in the community and to train physicians and nurses.

Wilson felt certain that given their history of generosity, local people would be willing to pitch in and help. The problem, Andrews informed the vice chancellor, was that Vanderbilt and the city of Nashville had historically been unable to get along, although he had to agree that a donor society was a good idea. Unfazed by the tradition of feuding, Wilson initiated the Canby Robinson Society, named after the man who had been the first dean of the Vanderbilt Medical School in 1920. Andrews stepped in as the society's first president.

"We called it an ambassadorship, a friendship," Andrews told *Vanderbilt Medicine* magazine. "It was not a project at that time to make money; it was a project to make friends."[29]

The Canby Robinson Society grew slowly but steadily, the recipient of donations from both within and outside the Medical Center. In time, it became a primary source for scholarships for deserving medical students. For Wilson, a by-product of the Canby Robinson Society was that it served as a brilliant public relations tactic. Wilson won over several local business leaders, who began taking his side during various fiery debates involving the hospital's construction, even as he was infuriating many Vanderbilt physicians.

Ed Nelson's appreciation of Vernon Wilson evolved over time. "Did you ever have one of those teachers who was so authoritative, so hard on you, and kept asking you to do things you were sure you couldn't do, and you couldn't wait to be done with that class?" he queried. "Then later, you realize that you have basic knowledge and skills that other people don't have—all because of that teacher. Suddenly, you start to hold that teacher in high regard. That's how it was with Vernon Wilson."[30]

On September 12, 1980, "under the glare of TV lights and the smiles of employees,"[31] all the Vanderbilt inpatients were moved from the aged hospital into the new 514-bed twin towers structure that was christened the new Vanderbilt University Hospital. A week later, an official dedication ceremony was held for the Vanderbilt Children's Hospital and Junior League Home under the guidance of Friends Chair Darlene Hoffman.

"We did it! And I mean 'we' in the most inclusive sense," gushed the Medical Center's PR chief, Kathryn Costello, who deemed the event a "smashing success."

"I am so thrilled to see the good effort that comes out of the combination of community and Vanderbilt people working together . . . [I]t is the joint effort that creates the best results."[32]

After the hoopla subsided, David Karzon walked the halls of the new Children's Hospital. What he'd initiated in 1970 as a clever marketing scheme, and spent a decade fighting for, building and developing had wound up as just another compromise—a hospital-within-a-hospital. As he surveyed the colorful walls, the brightly lit corridors, and the rooms with telephones and sleeper chairs, he began to realize that he could make this work. He might not have gotten what he'd asked for, but, ironically, he'd gotten what he wanted. The pediatric faculty would be right next door to the adult caregivers. Basic scientists and clinicians were so close in proximity that they could easily exchange ideas and collaborate on research projects. Because the two hospitals were sharing so many resources and so much equipment, the Medical Center would be saving enormous amounts of money.

Sure, he'd always said that Vanderbilt Children's Hospital was more than a place, more than geography, more than bricks and mortar. But as he surveyed his freshly opened unit, Karzon realized that bricks and mortar were actually integral to his dream—because they legitimized his dream. A new epoch of scientific discovery was just starting in 1980, and those on the forefront would open amazing frontiers in biomedical and biotechnological knowledge. Encased within Vanderbilt University Hospital, the Children's Hospital was poised to push itself right into the mix of globally significant research—and this time, without sacrificing patient care.

Already Karzon was pulling together a stellar team of clinicians and physician-scientists. And now, with his hardest days behind him, he felt confident that he also had the support of the local community.

Sixty years earlier, the polio epidemic had spawned the creation of the Junior League Home for Crippled Children and formed the roots of Vanderbilt Children's Hospital. David Karzon's early career was launched by efforts to find a vaccine for that disease. When Children's Hospital opened in 1980, it was a product of six decades of painstakingly rendered success. As a testament to that success, the new hospital did not include a polio ward. Thanks to the efforts of doctors like Amos Christie, Randy Batson, Pete Riley, David Karzon, and Mildred Stahlman; to surgeons, orthopedists, and politicians;

to physical therapists and occupational therapists; and to the financial and volunteer assistance from ordinary laypeople, medicine had advanced to the point where such a place, at last, was no longer needed.

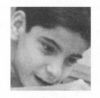

The Southern Dichotomy | 20

"We were feminists. Now we're out of style."

**—Mary Lee Manier,
Junior League president from 1960–62**

In October 1979, a year before the new hospital was to be completed, Vernon Wilson announced that he would be stepping down from his leadership role at the Medical Center as of June 1981. He was ready to retire, he told reporters, but he would see the construction of the new hospital through to the end. He didn't mention that he was battling heart disease and having significant health problems.

The announcement gave a search team headed by Dr. John Oates time to find the perfect candidate for what had suddenly become an extremely attractive position. The search team was scouting for somebody with high academic credentials, somebody who could carry Vanderbilt forward on its course of expansion.[1] The person they found was Dr. Roscoe "Ike" Robinson. He was everything Vernon Wilson was not—tall, eloquent, charming, warm, and immediately likeable. He also held a deep reverence for academic research and the role of physician-scientists. Not only that, Robinson also knew how to borrow money and float bonds for construction.

When Wilson retired, at his insistence, the Medical Center gave him no grand send-off, nor threw any parties of appreciation for his hard work and contributions. Only in 2002, ten years after his death, did Vanderbilt commission a portrait in his honor. His reign was so tempestuous, yet so crucial to Vanderbilt's growth, that many felt indebted to him only in hindsight.

245

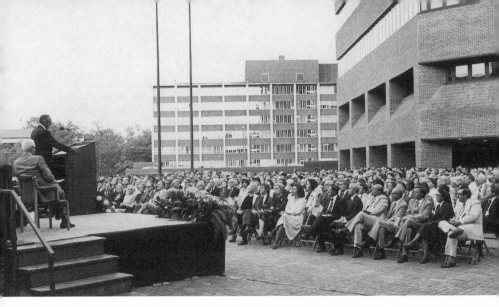

In September 1980, the new Vanderbilt University Hospital officially opened for business.

"Somebody had to die on the battlefield so we could get to the next step," admitted James O'Neill. "Vernon Wilson paved the way for the nice guy coming in."[2]

Which is one of the many lessons that emerged from the creation of Vanderbilt Children's Hospital. As lengthy and difficult as the process was, it was ultimately only a brief chapter in a larger story about a turbulent time in the life of a university during a turbulent point in American history; about a city trying to find its sea legs amid the waves of change; and about the people who were both catalysts for and catalyzed by the events around them.

The dichotomy found in this story reflects the ambivalence of the city itself. The archetypal Nashvillian has always been someone ready for a good fight while simultaneously yearning for conciliation. For example, John Seigenthaler remembered when he was editor of the *Tennessean* and Jimmy Stahlman was the all-powerful publisher of the rival *Banner*. On many days they would park their cars in adjacent parking lots and ride up the elevator together in the morning. Amon Evans, publisher of the *Tennessean*, was going through a bitter divorce at the time. "Glad to see you, son," Stahlman would say, "How's Amon doing?"

Seigenthaler would answer, "He's doing fine, Mr. Stahlman."

The *Banner* publisher, a man larger than life, would pull out his handkerchief and literally weep at the thought that Amon Evans was going through such a rough time.

"Well, give him my love, son," he'd say, patting Seigenthaler on the back.

Then the two men would step off the elevator, go to their respective offices, and spend the rest of the day in heated combat, each trying to bring the other man's newspaper to its knees.[3]

Categorizations and generalizations never fall neatly into place. As the president of the exclusive society of the Junior League, Mary Lee Manier led the charge for a children's hospital and the integration of the Home for Crippled Children long before either action was considered popular, or even appropriate in certain circles.

"We were feminists," she said in a Southern dialect that conjures up images not of burning bras and angry female marchers, but rather of sweet tea on the veranda, pillbox hats, and white driving gloves. "Now we're out of style."[4]

In fact, the dialect itself, spoken by so many of the people interviewed for this book, is going out of style. With its soft edges—even when spoken vehemently—it connotes a specific region of the South and a specific social echelon within that region. The grandchildren of these people, although equally Southern, educated, and refined, no longer speak that same dialect. Sadly, in a generation or two, it will likely be lost forever.

Part of the Southern dichotomy is the ability to see humor in the most serious of situations. Many years later, Carole Nelson still maintained that she made the right decision, the only decision she could make at the time, when she turned down Paul McCartney's offer to perform a benefit concert for the Children's Hospital.

She paused for a moment, a twinkle in her eye. An avid gardener, Nelson's lovely Belle Meade home is surrounded by beautiful landscaping and lush displays of flowers and trees. One day, around the same time that she was having to call off the dogs on the Paul McCartney concert, she heard a loud motorized sound coming from behind her house. Looking out her kitchen window, she saw that a Tennessee Bureau of Investigation helicopter had landed at the back of her property. She opened her back door and was met by her yardman, who stood before her with a quizzical smile on his face.

"What on earth is going on?" she asked him.

"That policeman is looking over your okra patch," the yardman said. "He thinks you're growing pot."

"So there you have it," Nelson said, aware of the poetic justice.

"Paul McCartney got arrested for marijuana, and I almost got arrested for okra."[5]

In the end, these small stories, these brief glimpses into Middle America provide the deepest insight into the unique forces that created a hospital for the region's children. Nobody wanted to give ground—neither the researchers at Vanderbilt nor the citizens of the town. Yet everybody wanted to help the children gain access to health care. That so much money was raised to found and support it and that so many movers and shakers placed their faith in a concept long before they had a building or a solid structure to rally behind, exemplifies the fabric of the people who live in Nashville.

But perhaps it is mail clerk William Ross, whose dollar launched the Palm Sunday Paper Sale every year, who best illustrates how Vanderbilt Children's Hospital came into being. Ross intuitively understood that although he could never give much, he could always give first—and it is in giving, first, that an individual makes an indelible, invaluable imprint on the lives of others.

The addition of the twin towers to the medical complex set a course for future growth and expansion for Vanderbilt University Medical Center.

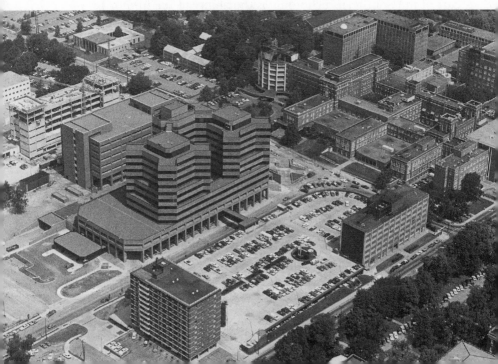

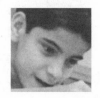

Epilogue

*"The atmosphere of the new hospital feels like a home,
which is what the originators of the Children's
Hospital were fighting for since the 1960s."*

**—Liza Lentz, former president of the
Junior League of Nashville**

From its humble beginnings as a noble concept, an ideal, and a tactic for gaining the interest and respect of the community, Vanderbilt Children's Hospital (VCH) has flourished and today is considered one of the top children's hospitals in the country. Thirty-five years from its inception, it is easy to see that the VCH forefathers and foremothers made the right call. As they predicted, the hospital has continued to function as a unifier of disparate factions within the local region. No matter where they stand on other issues, citizens tend to agree on the value and rectitude of providing outstanding health care to all children, regardless of their families' ability to pay.

After sixteen years as the vice chancellor for health affairs and having built up a world-class research enterprise, Ike Robinson stepped down in 1997 (he died in August 2004), and turned over the reins for running the multibillion-dollar Medical Center to his successor, Dr. Harry Jacobson.

One of Jacobson's first tasks was to begin preparing for the construction of a new, freestanding Vanderbilt Children's Hospital. James O'Neill recalled meeting with Jacobson several years earlier and promising him that, although building a new hospital would entail economic risks, Vanderbilt had the unprecedented opportunity

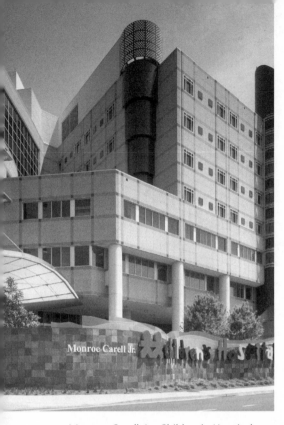

Monroe Carell Jr. Children's Hospital at Vanderbilt as it looks today. Photo by Scott McDonald/Hedrich Blessing.

to become the leading provider of pediatric care not only in the state of Tennessee, but in the entire Southeast. Jacobson liked that idea.

He called together consultants from national and local architecture firms. He set up commissions and advisory councils made up of doctors, nurses, business leaders, parents, and patients—all of whom, unlike in the past, had input into the construction of the new facility. They presented arguments about creating a nurturing atmosphere, about empowering parents, and about providing amenities that would make the hospital experience less traumatic for young patients—and this time those points of view fell on receptive ears.

From this group emerged a leader. Monroe Carell Jr., with the support of his wife, Ann, donated $25.6 million to the hospital and received naming rights. Carell also set to work spearheading a massive fund-raising campaign, personally making about seventy face-to-face calls on behalf of the project, and ultimately amassing $72.3 million in charitable gifts towards the new children's hospital. Fittingly, the first major donation was a $2 million gift from the Junior League of Nashville.

On February 8, 2004—twenty-four years after Vanderbilt Children's Hospital was incorporated within the twin towers building—a team of employees, students, and volunteers transferred more than one hundred pediatric patients from the fifth and sixth floors of Vanderbilt Hospital over to the resplendent, 616,000-square-foot, freestanding Monroe Carell Jr. Children's Hospital at Vanderbilt. The undependable sleeper chairs had long been laid to rest, as had the sterile, antiseptic ambiance. The rooms now include beds for parents, as well as desks, shelves, and storage space. The walls are decorated in bright colors and child-appropriate themes.

"The atmosphere of the new hospital feels like a home," commented Liza Lentz, "which is what the originators of the Children's Hospital were fighting for since the 1960s."[1]

Former Junior League president Joanne Bailey said triumphantly, "We kept fighting and it finally carried over."[2]

The freestanding Children's Hospital at Vanderbilt could never have happened were it not for a long line of people determined to increase the profile of pediatrics being practiced in Tennessee.

After he retired from the pediatric chairmanship in 1968, Amos Christie devoted much of his time to improving the delivery of health care to the underprivileged of Appalachia through the Vanderbilt Appalachian Student Health Coalition. In 1979, he received the John Howland Award, the highest honor granted by the American Pediatric Society. Throughout his years as a professor emeritus, Christie's relationship with Karzon never thawed, although Karzon continued to treat Christie with due respect and paid for his travel to seminars and ceremonies. Christie died in 1986 at the age of eighty-four. In 2005, the eighth floor of the doctors' office tower in the new stand-alone children's hospital was named in his honor.

As a fitting tribute, Robert Merrill wrote a memoir about his beloved mentor, *Amos Christie, M.D.: The Legacy of a Lineman*. Sadly, Merrill died of leukemia on January 11, 2006, while the book was in press.

Medical Affairs Dean Randy Batson left Vanderbilt in 1978 and spent the next eight years in Troy, Alabama, as president and physician-in-chief of the Charles Henderson Child Health Center, a public health care facility. He died on December 6, 2004, at the age of eighty-eight.

After eighteen years at the helm of the pediatrics department, having overseen a period of phenomenal growth both in patient load and research, David Karzon stepped down and returned to the laboratory, focusing on such devastating infectious diseases of children as HIV/AIDS. When Allaire retired from the Vanderbilt Law School in the mid-1990s, Karzon followed suit and retired as well. He and his wife now split their time between Nashville and a winter home in Tucson, Arizona.

In 1988, Ian Burr returned to the Medical Center and assumed the pediatric chairmanship. By this time, the hospital-within-a-hospital concept had gained wide acceptance, and scores of people from other regional medical centers across the country traveled to Vanderbilt to see how to implement a children's hospital within their own facilities. Under Burr's leadership, pediatrics grew to include twenty-nine subspecialties. By the late 1990s, with the plans for a large freestanding children's hospital under way, Burr stepped down as chairman and became associate vice chancellor for children's services. His primary job was to spend the next several years overseeing the design and development of the Monroe Carell Jr. Children's Hospital at Vanderbilt and the outpatient tower. He retired from Vanderbilt in 2006.

Dr. Arnold Strauss arrived at Vanderbilt in 2000 as the new chairman of pediatrics and the medical director of the Children's Hospital, offices he held until 2007.

James O'Neill had been recruited back to Vanderbilt during the 1990s to serve as the director of surgical sciences. Again, with the blueprints for the freestanding hospital in the drawing phase, he retired from that position in 2001 to assist in planning for the surgery section of the stand-alone Children's Hospital. In that endeavor, he once again solicited the aid of pediatric surgeon George Holcomb, who never relinquished the dream of such a hospital for the children of Middle Tennessee. Holcomb and O'Neill both remain professors of surgery emeritus at Vanderbilt University Medical Center.

The Monroe Carell Jr. Children's Hospital at Vanderbilt is a massive structure, operating at top capacity, with well over two hundred thousand patient visits each year. Among its assets are 216 inpatient beds, sixteen operating rooms, and a full-fledged pediatric emergency department that accepts patients from all over the world. In addition, the pediatric intensive care unit, originally funded by the Cook family as a tiny four-bed ward, has swelled to accommodate thirty-six patients. Within the first year of its move to the new freestanding facility, *Child Magazine* ranked VCH among the top children's hospitals in the country and named its childhood cancer program as one of the top ten pediatric cancer treatment centers in the nation. And thanks in part to the escalation of research at the Children's Hospital and to the leadership of Ike Robinson and Harry Jacobson, Vanderbilt University Medical Center has become the nation's fastest growing biomedical research institution in terms of grants funded by the National Institutes of Health.

Although their colleague Sarah Sell has retired from practicing medicine, Mildred Stahlman and Robert Cotton continue on the Vanderbilt faculty as members of the burgeoning Neonatal Intensive Care Unit team. Today, the NICU includes seventy-two beds—sixty in the Monroe Carell Jr. Hospital for transfer patients and twelve additional beds in the main hospital on the maternal-fetal unit. Throughout her career, Stahlman has accumulated numerous honors for her research, including the prestigious Virginia Apgar and John Howland Awards. In 2002, she was named Vanderbilt Medical Center Distinguished Alumna, and in 2004, received the same award from the university at large. The Angel emergency transport system, which she founded thirty years ago, still carries the most fragile babies to Vanderbilt from across the region.

Perhaps not surprisingly, many of those individuals and organizations that willed the Vanderbilt Children's Hospital into existence remain committed to the cause. Nelson Andrews, Ed Nelson, Pat Wilson, Alice Hooker, Fran Hardcastle, and Carole Nelson, to name a few, still play a major role in philanthropy devoted to benefit Vanderbilt. Into this mix has stepped the Ingram family, particularly Martha Ingram, the wife of Bronson, Hortense Ingram's now-deceased son. Bronson was also instrumental in backing the efforts of the Medical Center, as have been their children—Orrin, John, David, and Robin—all of whom have made tremendous personal and financial contributions to Vanderbilt University and its Medical Center.

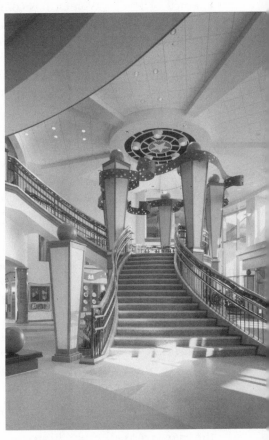

The lobby of the Monroe Carell Jr. Children's Hospital at Vanderbilt as it looks today. Photo by Craig Dugan/ Hedrich Blessing.

The Canby Robinson Society (CRS), begun on a wing and a prayer by Vernon Wilson, has evolved into one of the city's most dynamic philanthropic societies. With an original membership of 189 in 1980, it now includes close to 4,000 individuals, who in 2005 raised $14 million in charitable gifts. A portion of CRS philanthropy is devoted to full-tuition scholarships to support the training of medical students and MD/PhD students.

Over a stretch of decades, the Nashville section of the National Council of Jewish Women has continued its dedication to local civic causes. Likewise, the Friends of Vanderbilt Children's Hospital has expanded from its infancy with eight founding members into a collection of over two thousand civic-minded men and women operating in five counties in Middle Tennessee and Kentucky. The Friends organization raises millions of charitable dollars each year to promote the health of area children.

By the same token, the Junior League of Nashville has never wavered in its faithfulness towards improving the lives of local children, an issue it has held dear since 1923. Comprised of nearly two thousand women of all races, creeds, and colors, it is the tenth largest league in the Association of Junior Leagues International, and has provided ongoing funding for the Junior League Family Resource Center, the Child Life program, and various other programs and projects (amounting to $450,000 in 2005 alone) at the freestanding Children's Hospital. The Home Board remains an integral part of the local Junior League, and the Trust Fund, protected by decree of the supreme court of the state of Tennessee, has now blossomed into millions of dollars designated to serve the area's youngest and neediest citizens.

Middle Tennessee is an extraordinary, quirky place and its citizens have a distinct appreciation for the milieu in which they reside. Nothing is ever clear-cut. In the 1960s, *Banner* publisher Jimmy Stahlman, for example, opposed the lunch counter sit-ins; however, he was a loyal and steadfast supporter of Mayor Ben West, even after the mayor agreed to integrate the local lunch counters. City leaders favored building a children's hospital but would not embark on that mission unless Vanderbilt consented to the terms. Ladies of the National Jewish Council and the Junior League believed they should open their respective convalescent homes to black children, but grappled with how to do so gracefully and graciously.

Because their arch-rival newspapers were disputing every point in every discussion, Nashvillians had no excuse for being complacent or unaware during this era. Stahlman and his nemesis/friend John

Seigenthaler from the *Tennessean* understood the power of the press and they used it to push their agendas forward.

James Stahlman died in 1976 at a meeting of the Vanderbilt Board of Trust. Fellow board member Pat Wilson recalled that Stahlman had stood up to make a point and was pointing and gesticulating when he suddenly collapsed to the floor. "I liked Jimmy," Wilson said. "I hardly ever agreed with him, but I still liked him."

In 1991, John Seigenthaler retired as chairman emeritus from the *Tennessean* to establish the Freedom Forum First Amendment Center at Vanderbilt University, over which he continues to preside. In 1998, the Gannett Corporation, parent company of the *Tennessean*, purchased the *Banner* newspaper and shut down the afternoon daily for good. The death of the *Banner* signaled the end of a century and a half in which local citizens were never permitted the luxury of ennui, because their homegrown newspapers forced them, rightly or wrongly, to care.

Time has also transformed Vanderbilt University's perspective on its role in local history. The Reverend James Lawson, who had been expelled from the Divinity School during the sit-ins, has since been recognized as valiant champion of the rights of the disenfranchised. In 2005, he was named Vanderbilt Distinguished Alumnus and now serves as an esteemed adjunct professor in the same Divinity School from which he was dismissed decades earlier.

It seems that Nashville has always been caught in the twilight between progress and preservation. From that novel position has emerged a unique culture of generosity and trust, tempered by wariness. Knowing full well that they were part of the game, the city's leaders, male and female, supported and convinced others to join them in supporting a virtual children's hospital embedded within Vanderbilt Hospital. In a period of political turmoil and medical innovation, decision-makers deliberately bought into the hospital-within-a-hospital concept, realizing that it would allow them to step carefully into shifting sands. Having made that commitment, they spent the next decade investing in and working on the project with dogged enthusiasm, thereby giving it legitimacy.

Middle Tennessee now awaits the emergence of a new generation of young, undaunted leaders—people willing to fight for the poor, the sick, and the young; people willing to give of their hard-earned dollars because they believe that it is their responsibility to improve their community; people who refuse to be thwarted by convoluted logistics and political barriers.

While working on this book and interviewing the many individuals involved in the founding of the Vanderbilt Children's Hospital, one common refrain kept cropping up to the question, "Why did you keep pursuing a children's hospital after so many setbacks?"

Time and time again, the interviewees would shrug their shoulders and answer, "Because it was the right thing to do."

Notes

Chapter 1

1. *Tennessee Blue Book, 2001–2004* (online version), 394–410, http://www.state.tn.us/sos/bluebook/online/bbonline.htm.
2. Ibid.
3. *Tennessee Encyclopedia of History and Culture*, s.v. "Vanderbilt University" (by Patricia Miletich), http://160.36.208.47/FMPro?-db=tnencyc&-format=tdetail.htm.
4. James Summerville, *Nashville Medicine: A History* (Birmingham, Ala: Association Publishing Company, 1999), 43. Quote attributed to Daniel Drake.
5. Ibid.
6. Amos Christie, MD, "Early History of Medical Education in Nashville," *Journal of the Tennessee Medical Assn.* 62:9 (1969): 819–829.
7. Dr. Owen H. Wilson would also become godfather to Mildred Stahlman, a pioneering neonatologist, who figures prominently in the history of Vanderbilt Children's Hospital.
8. The formal name for the Flexner Report was "Medical Education in the United States and Canada."
9. Mark Silverman, T. Jock Murray, Charles S. Bryan, eds., *The Quotable Osler* (Philadelphia, Penn: American College of Physicians, 2003), 47.
10. Ibid., 44.
11. Summerville, *Nashville Medicine: A History*, 45.
12. Vanderbilt Medical Center School of Medicine. "History of the Medical School," http://www.mc.Vanderbilt.edu/medschool/history.php.
13. Summerville, *Nashville Medicine: A History*, 46–49. Note: The only other black medical school Flexner suggested remain open was the one at Howard University in Washington, D.C.
14. Christie, "Early History of Medical Education in Nashville," 819–829.

Chapter 2

1. "The Junior League History: Critical Milestones in the Movement," The Association of Junior Leagues International, Inc., http://www.ajli.org/?nd=history.
2. Ibid.
3. Hattie Stuart, ed., "The Junior League Home" (Nashville, Tenn.: Junior League of Nashville, 1983), 3.
4. Ibid., 2.
5. "In the Beginning," adapted from "The Junior League Home" and from the Junior League's first community magazine, *The Volunteer* (Fall 1981): 2.
6. Mary Lee Bartlett, president, Junior League of Nashville, 2005–2006, personal interview, March 31, 2005.
7. Kent Ewing Ballow, phone interview, July 7, 2005. Note: Following in the footsteps of her grandmother, Kent Ewing Ballow served as the 2001–2002 president of the Junior League of Nashville.
8. Ibid.
9. "The Junior League Home," 2.
10. Mary Stahlman Douglas (with additions), "A History of the Junior League of Nashville," (Nashville, Tenn.: Junior League of Nashville, n.d.), 108. From the files of Missy Scoville.
11. "The Junior League Home," 13.
12. Mary Lee Bartlett.
13. "The Junior League Home," 13.
14. Carole Bucy, "Tennessee Women and the Vote: Tennessee's Pivotal Role in the Passage of the Nineteenth Amendment" (Written for the seventy-fifth anniversary of the ratification of the Nineteenth Amendment), 1995, http://www2.vscc.cc.tn.us/cbucy/History%202030/suffrage.htm.
15. Ibid.
16. Ibid. To clarify, that was Nashville's *white* contingent. African American women, led by Frankie J. Pierce, were fighting just as desperately for passage of the Nineteenth Amendment.
17. Ibid.
18. Ibid. The note from Harry Burns's mother read: "Dear Son: Hurrah and vote for suffrage! I noticed some of the speeches against. I have been watching to see how you stood but have not notices [*sic*] anything. Don't forget to be a good boy and help . . . put the 'rat' in ratification. Your Mother."
19. Liza Beazley Lentz, personal interview, April 6, 2005. Lentz was Junior League of Nashville president, 1995–96.
20. Cornelia Keeble and Anne Dallas Dudley traveled in the same elite social circles and Dudley was an early member of the Junior League of Nashville. According to the June 1926 issue of the *Junior League Bulletin*, published by the organization's national headquarters, Anne Dallas Dudley hosted one of the resplendent dinners when the national conference was held in Nashville.
21. Mary Stahlman Douglas, 108.
22. Ibid.
23. In May of 1926, 666 delegates from Junior League affiliates gathered in Nashville for the national conference, headed by local president, Frances Dudley Brown. In addition to the business and meetings, the delegates were treated to a seated dinner for 600 at the home of the Rogers Caldwells, dancing at the Belle Meade Country Club, a presidents' luncheon at the Hermitage Hotel (where, by the way, both the pro- and anti-suffragists had set up headquarters over the Nineteenth Amendment in 1920), and a trip to Louisville for the running of the Kentucky Derby. *The Parrot* (Nov.–Dec. 1962): 10. From the personal scrapbook of Mary Louise Tidwell.
24. Kent Ewing Ballow.

25. Junior League of Nashville 1962 Provisional Training Course, Oct. 15–Nov. 9. From the scrapbook of Mary Louise Tidwell.

26. In 2006, the criteria for membership are not as stringent. Members are no longer forced to sustain at age forty, but instead are asked to devote a minimum of five years of active service no matter their age or when they became active members. The rules for selecting members have also been relaxed to enable women of various social classes, races, and religions to join.

27. Mary Lee Bartlett.

28. Mary Louise Tidwell, personal interview, April 13, 2005.

29. Ibid. Ann McLemore Harwell was Junior League of Nashville president from 1946–47, 1947–58.

30. Martha Rivers Ingram, *E. Bronson Ingram: Complete These Unfinished Tasks of Mine* (Franklin, Tenn.: Hillsboro Press, 2001), 10. Note: Hortense Bigelow Ingram's father was president of the St. Paul Fire and Marine Insurance Company.

31. Alice Ingram Hooker, daughter of Hortense and Hank Ingram, personal interview, June 14, 2005.

32. Kent Ewing Ballow.

33. Alice Ingram Hooker.

34. Ibid.

35. Ibid.

36. Ibid.

37. Mary Schlater Stumb, personal interview, April 14, 2005. Stumb was president of the Junior League of Nashville during the 1971–72 term.

Chapter 3

1. "The Junior League Home," 18.

2. Mary Stahlman Douglas.

3. Ibid.

4. In fact, Jimmy Stahlman became potentate of the Al Menah Shrine Temple in 1937.

5. *Pyramid Shriners,* "Shrine History," http://www.pyramidshriners.com/history.htm.

6. "The Shrine of North America," http://shrineauditorium.com/shriners.html.

7. Ibid.

8. "Al Menah History," http://www.almenahshriners.org/history.htm.

9. http://shrineauditorium.com/shriners.html.

10. "Selections from the Diaries of Lucius E. Burch, M.D., 1921–1938," March 27, 1921, Vanderbilt Historical Collection, Eskind Biomedical Library.

11. "Shriners Hospitals for Children," http://www.shrinershq.org/shc/lexington/index.html.

12. Suzanne Windorfer, administrative assistant for Al Menah Shriners since 1967, phone interview, July 21, 2005.

13. "The Junior League Home," 18.

14. Mary Stahlman Douglas.

15. "The *Tennessean,*" http://www.answers.com/main/ntquery?tname=the%2Dtennessean&print=true.

16. Don H. Doyle, *Nashville Since the 1920s* (Knoxville, Tenn.: University of Tennessee Press, 1985), 87.

17. Willy Stern, "Grading the Daily, Part 1—The Way Things Were," *Nashville Scene* (April 26–May 1, 2001).

18. Leon Alligood, "End of Story," *Nashville Banner,* February 20, 1998, sec. A-2.

19. John Seigenthaler, former publisher of the *Tennessean,* personal interview, April 19, 2005.

20. Kent Ewing Ballow.

21. Frances Hardcastle, president of the Junior League of Nashville, 1975–76, personal interview, April 20, 2005.

22. "The Junior League Home," 18.

23. Mary Ann Johns, polio survivor, comments excerpted from *Junior League of Nashville: Celebrating 80 Years,* video (Nashville, Tenn.: Junior League of Nashville), 2002.

24. Mary Stahlman Douglas.

25. Frances Jackson, president of the Junior League of Nashville, 1969–70; chair of the Junior League Home Board, 1980–81, personal interview, April 20, 2005.

26. Wilson "Woody" Sims, attorney at law, personal interview, April 21, 2005.

27. Junior League of Nashville, "In the Beginning," flyer (Nashville, Tenn.: Junior League of Nashville, n.d.).

28. "The Junior League Home," 3–4.

29. "In the Beginning."

30. Nickie Lancaster, polio survivor, phone interview, April 18, 2005. Lancaster went on to receive her nursing degree and is currently the coordinator of the Polio Heroes of Tennessee support group for the Easter Seals Society of Tennessee.

31. Justine Milam, phone interview, April 1, 2005.

32. Nickie Lancaster.

33. Mary Ann Johns.

34. Nickie Lancaster.

35. Helen Clark, polio survivor, comments excerpted from *Junior League of Nashville: Celebrating 80 Years,* 2002.

Chapter 4

1. Obituary, in *The Child,* "Dr. Horton Casparis, Physician to Children," December 1942, http://hearth.library.cornell.edu/cgi/t/test/pageviewer-idx?c91bd2f4217e2ba702b37721521a4e4&idno=4732639_155_009&c=hearth&view=im.

2. Amos Christie, *As I Remember It* (self-published, February 1971), 3–6.

3. Dr. William DeLoache, pediatrician and graduate of Vanderbilt Medical School, phone interview, April 18, 2005. On the other hand, DeLoache added, in those days medical personnel had to be in the patients' rooms nearly all the time. This was before the invention of the IV, and many

children were admitted with infectious dysentery. "We had to push fluids 'round the clock—every four hours," he said.

4. Paul K. Conkin, *Gone with the Ivy: A Biography of Vanderbilt University* (Knoxville, Tenn.: University of Tennessee Press, 1985), 421.

5. Harvie Branscomb, Chancellor Emeritus, Vanderbilt University, Nashville, Tennessee. Excerpted from "The Christie Era," remarks given by the Amos Christie Symposium, Sept. 19, 1987.

6. Christie, *As I Remember It*, 7.

7. Ibid., 8.

8. Ibid.

9. Dr. Harris "Pete" Riley. Professor of pediatrics, Vanderbilt University Medical School, personal interview, June 6, 2005.

10. Christie, *As I Remember It*, 8–11.

11. Ibid., 11.

12. William DeLoache.

13. Dr. Sarah Sell, personal interview, April 28, 2005. "Katie Dodd was a Spartan, but everybody loved her. She was a fantastic teacher," Sell said. Dodd and her nieces would go swimming in the Cumberland River every Sunday, no matter the weather. In the winter they'd push the ice around to make room for them to swim.

14. Christie, *As I Remember It*, 13.

15. Ibid.

16. Ibid.

17. Bill Snyder, "Intensive Caring: Stahlman Has Always Demanded Excellence from Herself, Others," VUMC *Reporter* (Feb. 4, 2005): 1, 3–4.

18. Ibid.

19. Dr. Mildred Stahlman, personal interview with Dr. David Karzon, late 1990s.

20. Mildred Stahlman, excerpted from transcript of personal interview with Bill Snyder, 2005.

21. Sarah Sell.

22. Ibid.

23. Ibid.

24. Dr. Stuart Finder, PhD, director of the Center for Clinical and Research Ethics at Vanderbilt University Medical Center, personal interview, April 5, 2005.

25. Ibid.

26. Those discoveries include the chicken embryo technique for the production of vaccines; the understanding that fowlpox contained infectious viral particles; the recognition that mumps is caused by a virus; insights into the pathophysiology of the circulatory system; and findings that determined histoplasmosis to be a fungal infection.

27. Dr. William Wadlington, professor of pediatrics at Vanderbilt University School of Medicine, phone interview, August 19, 2005.

28. As a testament to the excellence of the training received by members of the department, some ten or so pediatricians who trained under Christie went on to chair pediatric departments across the country, as well as to hold some of the most prestigious positions within the most powerful pediatric associations.

This is a remarkable achievement, particularly given how small the Vanderbilt pediatric department was and how few people trained there.

29. Dr. Robert Merrill, professor of pediatrics, Vanderbilt School of Medicine, personal interview, May 17, 2005.

30. Ibid.

31. Ibid.

32. Dr. William Altemeier, professor of pediatrics, phone interview, June 20, 2005.

33. Harris Riley.

34. Robert Merrill.

35. Ibid; Dr. Floyd W. Denny, Department of Pediatrics, University of North Carolina School of Medicine at Chapel Hill, North Carolina, excerpted from "Premier Gathering of the Friends of Amos Christie, Light Hall, Vanderbilt University, Nashville, Tennessee," Sept. 19, 1987.

36. Ibid; Dr. Eric Chazen, pediatrician, phone interview, June 15, 2005.

37. Christie, *As I Remember It*, 25.

38. Mrs. Bennie Batson, wife of former pediatrician and Dean of Medicine Randy Batson, phone interview, June 2, 2005.

39. Christie, *As I Remember It*, 49–50.

40. Robert Merrill.

41. Bennie Batson.

42. Robert Merrill.

43. Linda Christie Williams Moynihan, daughter of Amos Christie. Personal interview, May 9, 2005.

44. Ibid; Sarah Sell; Bennie Batson; Christie, *As I Remember It*, 26; Amos Christie, personal correspondence with Chancellor Harvie Branscomb, June 14, 1985; Robert Merrill.

45. Robert Merrill.

46. Christie, *As I Remember It*, 26.

Chapter 5

1. Lisa A. DuBois, "Ernest Goodpasture and the Mass Production of Vaccines," *Lens: A New Way of Looking at Science* (Vanderbilt University Medical Center, Spring 2004): 26. Goodpasture's chick embryo technique for growing massive quantities of vaccine is still being used in the twenty-first century.

2. Stuart Finder.

3. Dr. Robert D. Collins, "Troubled Times, 1945–50," *Ernest William Goodpasture: Scientist, Scholar, Gentleman* (Franklin, Tenn.: Hillsboro Press, 2002), 210, 220.

4. Ibid., 215.

5. Ibid., 219–220.

6. Ibid., 218. The fund's name was later changed to the more decorous "Emergency Hospital Fund."

7. Christie, *As I Remember It*, 54–55.

8. Amos Christie, "Report of the Committee on the Financial Crisis of the Vanderbilt University School of Medicine and Hospital," December 30, 1948.

9. Conkin, *Gone with the Ivy*, 494–95.

10. Ibid.

11. Christie, "Report of the Committee on the Financial Crisis of the Vanderbilt University School of Medicine and Hospital."

12. Collins, "Troubled Times," 229.

13. Ibid., 231.

14. Robert Merrill.

15. Ibid.

16. Christie, "Report of the Committee on the Financial Crisis of the Vanderbilt University School of Medicine and Hospital."

17. Sarah Sell.

18. Eric Chazen.

19. Dr. James O'Neill, former director of Surgical Services at Vanderbilt University Medical School, phone interview, April 26, 2005.

20. Robert D. Collins.

Chapter 6

1. Lisa A. DuBois, "Polio: The Fight Continues," *Lens: A New Way of Looking at Science* (Vanderbilt University Medical Center, Spring 2004): 25.

2. Christie, *As I Remember It*, 26; Nickie Lancaster.

3. Marjorie Mathias Dobbs, former nurse at Vanderbilt Hospital. Excerpted from "Some Memories of the Polio Days," from the files of Nickie Lancaster of the Polio Heroes of Tennessee Support Group for Easter Seals of Tennessee, Sept. 30, 1989.

4. Ibid.

5. Nickie Lancaster.

6. Marjorie Mathias Dobbs.

7. Sarah Sell.

8. "No Child Is Ever Alone" *Nashville Tennessean Magazine* (January 15, 1950): 13–14.

9. Christie, *As I Remember It*, 26–27.

10. Ibid.

11. Joan Armour, "Tank Town: Its Inhabitants: Polio Patients at Vanderbilt," *Nashville Tennessean Magazine* (January 23, 1955).

12. Marjorie Mathias Dobbs.

13. Joan Armour.

14. Marjorie Mathias Dobbs.

15. "No Child Is Ever Alone."

16. Nelson Andrews, president of Brookside Properties, personal interview, April 7, 2005.

17. "No Child Is Ever Alone," 13–14.

18. When Percie Warner Lea came in to the newspaper office wanting to talk about her March of Dimes press releases, said former *Tennessean* publisher John Seigenthaler, the reporters stood up—and those crusty, hotshot journalists rarely stood for anyone. "Mrs. Lea was treated with great deference and great respect," he said.

19. Deborah Kinsman, physical therapist, personal correspondence from the files of Nickie Lancaster of the Polio Heroes of Tennessee Support Group.

20. Dorothy Fredrickson, physical therapist, personal correspondence from the files of Nickie Lancaster of the Polio Heroes of Tennessee Support Group.

21. Ibid.

22. Nickie Lancaster.

23. James O'Neill.

24. Ibid.

25. Ross Fitzgerald, "5,000 Parents to Fight Polio in Jan. 21 'Lights-On' Drive," *Nashville Banner* (Dec. 19, 1951).

26. Christie, *As I Remember It*, 27.

27. John Simmons, *The Scientific 100: A Ranking of the Most Influential Scientists, Past and Present* (New York: Citadel Press, 1996), 425–429; "The 50th Anniversary Program," http://www.polio.umich.edu/program, April 12, 2005.

28. Harris Riley.

29. "Citations for Dr. Jonas E. Salk and The National Foundation for Infantile Paralysis for the Polio Vaccine," http://www.classbrain.com/artteenest/publish/printer_citation_polio_vaccine.shtml.

30. Lewis Williams and Sarah Cash, "Polio Still Strikes Many; 4 Lawrence Countians Ill" *Nashville Banner* (June 26, 1959).

31. "3 More Children Struck by Polio: New Cases Bring Total to 80 in State, More Than Double '58 Figure" *Tennessean* (August 20, 1959).

32. Christie, *As I Remember It*, 27.

33. Robert Merrill.

Chapter 7

1. "Study of The Junior League Home for Crippled Children," conducted by the Home Administration Board, under Chairman Mary Louise Lea Tidwell, 1957–58. From the personal files of Mary Louise Tidwell.

2. Chorea is a term for a number of central nervous system disorders marked by jerky, spasmodic movements of the arms, legs, trunk, and face.

3. Elizabeth Jacobs, former president of the Nashville Section of the National Council of Jewish Women, phone interview, September 7, 2005.

4. Ibid.

5. Leah Rose Werthan, former chair of the Nashville Section of the Council of Jewish Women's Home for Convalescent Care, "Special Oral History Project: Past Presidents." Interviewed by Dianne D. Gilbert, May 27, 1988. From the Archives of the Jewish Federation of Nashville and Middle Tennessee.

6. Press release from the National Council of Jewish Women, issued from New York, September 7, 1947. From the Archives of the Jewish Federation of Nashville and Middle Tennessee.

7. Leah Rose Werthan.

8. Feodora S. Frank, *Five Families and Eight Young Men (Nashville and her Jewry, 1850–1861)* (Nashville, Tenn.: Tennessee Book Company, 1962), 39.

9. *A Caring Community: The History of the Jews in Nashville*, video (Nashville, Tenn.: Jewish Federation of Nashville and Middle Tennessee, 2003).

10. Mid-Missouri Civil War Round Table, "Another Order No. 11: A Near-American Holocaust of 1862," http://www.mmcwrt.org/2001/default0104.htm.

11. "General Grant's Infamy," Jewish Virtual Library, http://www.jewishvirtuallibrary.org/jsource/anti-semitism/grant.html.

12. Feodora S. Frank, *Beginnings on Market Street (Nashville and her Jewry, 1861–1901)* (Nashville, Tenn.: Jewish Community of Nashville and Middle Tennessee 1976), 91.

13. *A Caring Community: The History of the Jews in Nashville*, video.

14. Resolution No. RS2001-721, "A resolution recognizing the 100-Year Anniversary of the National Council of Jewish Women (NCJW), Nashville Section," http://www.nashville.gov/mc/resolutions/prev/rs2001_721.htm.

15. *A Caring Community: The History of the Jews in Nashville*, video.

16. Leah Rose Werthan.

17. Press release from the National Council of Jewish Women, September 7, 1947. From the Archives of the Jewish Federation of Nashville and Middle Tennessee.

18. Leah Rose Werthan.

19. Ibid.

20. Press release from the National Council of Jewish Women, September 7, 1947; *The Red Feather Show*, transcript of radio show, June 8, 1952, 10:00 p.m., Station WMAK. From the Archives of the Jewish Federation of Nashville and Middle Tennessee.

21. Minutes from the Council's Administrative Board meeting, February 12, 1957. From the Archives of the Jewish Federation of Nashville and Middle Tennessee.

22. Elizabeth Jacobs.

23. Virginia Bivin, "Minister Lauds Jewish Women's Efforts in Maintenance of Children's Home Here," *Nashville Banner*, June 10, 1952.

24. Amos Christie, personal letter to Mrs. Jonas and Mrs. Cohen, December 12, 1953. From the Archives of the Jewish Federation of Nashville and Middle Tennessee; Amos Christie, excerpt of letter to the National Council of Jewish Women (NCJW), included in "Self-Evaluation Study of the Council Home for Convalescent Children," 1954. From the Archives of the Jewish Federation of Nashville and Middle Tennessee.

25. Christie, "Self-Evaluation Study."

26. Dana Pride, "The Great Divide," *Nashville: An American Self-Portrait*, eds. John Edgerton and E. Thomas Wood (Nashville, Tenn.: Beaten Biscuit Press, 2001), 245–254.

27. Minutes from the Council's Executive Board meetings, March 13, 1956; April 10, 1956; June 19, 1956. From the Archives of the Jewish Federation of Nashville and Middle Tennessee.

28. Draft of letter from the Nashville Section to the National Council of Jewish Women, undated. From the Archives of the Jewish Federation of Nashville and Middle Tennessee.

29. Ibid.

30. Doyle, *Nashville Since the 1920s*, 242; "Jewish Center Blasted," *Tennessean* (March 17, 1958): 1.

31. Minutes of the Executive Committee of the NCJW, May 13, 1958. From the Archives of the Jewish Federation of Nashville and Middle Tennessee.

32. Minutes of the Executive Committee of the NCJW, September 9, 1958; October 14, 1958; November 18, 1958. From the Archives of the Jewish Federation of Nashville and Middle Tennessee.

33. Louise Katzman, former president of the Nashville section of the National Council of Jewish Women, phone interview, June 15, 2005; Elizabeth Jacobs.

Chapter 8

1. Sarah Sell.

2. Ibid.

3. Conkin, *Gone with the Ivy*, 516–518.

4. Mary Stumb. Mrs. Stumb also related this story: In 1981, Ike Robinson was named the vice chancellor for medical affairs at Vanderbilt. Shortly after he arrived, a delegation from the Junior League showed up at his office and said, "Dr. Robinson, now here's what you're going to do . . ." Robinson, who had a wry, self-deprecating sense of humor, would later recount that first meeting. He said that when he got to Vanderbilt and was holding such an important position, everybody paid him such deference. He thought he was pretty hot stuff—that is, until the ladies of the Junior League showed up and started bossing him around, putting him in his place!

5. The following passage about the racial unrest in the 1960s is an interpretation and synopsis of events gleaned from the following sources: Ridley Wills, historian, personal interview, April 7, 2005; Don H. Doyle, *Nashville Since the 1920s* (Knoxville, Tenn.: University of Tennessee Press, 1985); Paul K. Conkin, *Gone with the Ivy: A Biography of Vanderbilt University* (Knoxville, Tenn.: University of Tennessee Press, 1985); David Halberstam, *The Children* (New York: Random House, 1998); John Lewis, *Walking with the Wind* (New York: Simon & Schuster, 1998); Amos Christie, *As I Remember It* (self-published, 1971); Bill Carey, *Chancellors, Commodores, & Coeds* (Nashville, Tenn.: Clearbrook Press Publishing, 2003); Ray Waddle, "Days of Thunder: The Lawson Affair," *Vanderbilt Magazine* (Fall 2002).

6. Conkin, *Gone with the Ivy*, 552.

7. Sarah Sell.

8. Christie, *As I Remember It*, 47.

9. Ridley Wills, Tennessee historian, personal interview, April 7, 2005.

10. Amos Christie, personal correspondence to Chancellor Harvie Branscomb, June 24, 1985.

11. Joanne Bailey, president of the Junior League of Nashville, 1967–68, personal interview, April 6, 2005.

12. Frances Jackson.

13. Mary Lee Manier, president of the Junior League of Nashville, 1960–61, 1961–62, personal interview, April 6, 2005.

14. Minutes of Junior League Board Meeting, November 9, 1960. From the Archives of the Junior League of Nashville.

15. "Study of the Junior League Home for Crippled Children," conducted by the Home Administration Board, 1957–58. From the personal files of Mary Louise Tidwell.

16. Ibid.

17. Mary Lee Manier; Minutes of Junior League Board Meeting, December 1960. From the Archives of the Junior League of Nashville.

18. Proposal: "Plan for Admitting Negro Patients to the Junior League Home for Crippled Children," Minutes of Junior League Board Meeting, November 9, 1960. From the Archives of the Junior League of Nashville.

19. Personal correspondence from Mrs. Walter M. "Dudley" Morgan, chair, Administration Committee, Junior League of Nashville, to Cromwell Tidwell, DDS. From the personal files of Mary Louise Tidwell.

Chapter 9

1. Dr. George Holcomb, pediatric surgeon, personal interview, April 25, 2005.

2. "History of Children's Hospitals," from the National Association of Children's Hospitals and Related Institutions (NACHRI) and National Association of Children's Hospitals (NACH) Web page, http://www.childrenshospitals.net/Template .cfm?Section=Home&CONTENTID=7418&TEM PLATE=/ContentManagement/ContentDisplay.cfm.

3. "Mission and History," Children's Hospital of Philadelphia Web page, http://www.chop.edu/ about_chop/mission_hist.shtml.

4. "History of Children's Hospitals."

5. James O'Neill, personal correspondence to Dr. Harris D. Riley, MD, June 24, 1999. From the personal files of James O'Neill.

6. "About Dr. J. William Hillman," from the Vanderbilt Orthopedic Web page, http://www.mc .vanderbilt.edu/ortho/hillman1.html.

7. James O'Neill, personal interview, April 26, 2005.

8. Christie, *As I Remember It*, 25.

9. George Holcomb, "Children's Memorial Community Hospital, Nashville," speech and proposal, 1961. From the personal files of Dr. George Holcomb.

10. Hydrocephalus is a congenital disease caused by an abnormal increase in the cerebrospinal fluid around the brain, resulting in the enlargement of the head because the bones of the skull are unfused.

11. Beth Odle, former patient at the Nashville Junior League Home for Crippled Children, phone interview, May 30, 2005.

12. George Holcomb and information from personal files of George Holcomb.

13. George Holcomb, "Children's Memorial Community Hospital, Nashville," speech and proposal, 1961.

14. George Holcomb, personal correspondence to Mr. W. H. Criswell, July 21, 1961. From the personal files of George Holcomb.

15. Alice Ingram Hooker.

16. Ibid.

17. Christie, *As I Remember It*, 93.

18. "Statement of Belief As Concerns A Children's Hospital for Nashville." From the personal files of George Holcomb.

19. Jack Setters, "Dr. Sanger Cautions Against Hasty Move On Children's Hospital," *Nashville Banner* (September 19, 1961).

20. Dr. Addison Scoville, personal report entitled: "To Discuss the Proposal of a Children's Hospital," July 7, 1961. From the personal files of George Holcomb.

21. Conkin, *Gone with the Ivy*, 497–498.

22. George Holcomb.

23. Mary Lee Manier.

24. James O'Neill.

25. Addison Scoville.

26. Ibid.

27. George Holcomb, personal correspondence to Amos Christie, July 7, 1961. From the personal files of George Holcomb.

28. Amos Christie, personal correspondence to George Holcomb, July 8, 1961. From the personal files of George Holcomb.

29. Ibid.

30. Ibid.

31. Jack Setters, "Vanderbilt's Children's Hospital Is Already Under Construction: Need For Another Facility Being Questioned By Many," *Nashville Banner* (July 26, 1961).

32. Jack Setters, "Torrence Says City Cannot Help Finance Children's Hospital," *Nashville Banner* (July 27, 1961).

33. Jack Setters. "Dr. Sanger Cautions Against Hasty Move."

34. Ibid.

35. Editorial, "Dr. Sanger Warns Against Leap In The Dark," *Nashville Banner* (October 9, 1961).

36. George Holcomb, personal letter to Addison Scoville Jr. From the personal files of George Holcomb.

37. Ibid. *Banner* publisher James Stahlman's daughter Mildred was a member of the Vanderbilt pediatric faculty and Stahlman was a university trustee.

38. Ibid.

39. Julie Hollabaugh, "Massey Heads Hospital Group," *Tennessean* (February 1962).

40. Robert Merrill.

41. Eric Chazen.

42. Sarah Sell.

43. Christie, *As I Remember It*, 25.

Chapter 10

1. Dr. Thomas Graham, former chief of pediatric cardiology at Vanderbilt University Medical Center, personal interview, April 11, 2005.

2. Hyaline membrane disease, or respiratory distress syndrome, is caused by a lack of the substance in the lungs of premature infants, leading to the collapse of the lung alveoli. "You hardly see hyaline membrane disease anymore, because you can give surfactant by inhalation and prevent or minimize it in most cases," Graham said. "Today Patrick Bouvier Kennedy would be a drop-kick [success story]. He'd only be in the hospital two or three weeks and then he'd go home."

3. "Patrick Bouvier Kennedy," http://www.patrick-bouvier-kennedy.biography.ms/.

4. Mildred Stahlman, from transcript of personal interview with David Karzon, undated.

5. Ann Stahlman Hill was a pioneer in her own right, serving as one of the leaders in the national children's theater movement. As a result of her efforts, Nashville Children's Theatre has long been regarded as one of the leading children's theater companies in America.

6. Billy J. Slate, "Nashville on the High Seas," http://pages.prodigy.net/nhn.slate/nh00032.html.

7. Mildred Stahlman; Bill Snyder, "Intensive Caring: Stahlman Has Always Demanded Excellence From Herself, Others." VUMC *Reporter* (February 4, 2005; "Inventory of Stahlman, Mildred Thornton (1922–) Collection Number 382." http://www.mc.vanderbilt.edu/sc_diglib/archColl/382.html; Sarah Sell.

8. Dr. John Lukens, former chief of pediatric hematology/oncology at Vanderbilt University Medical Center, personal interview, September 13, 2005.

9. Dr. Ian Burr, former chairman of pediatrics at Vanderbilt University Hospital, personal interview, April 8, 2005.

10. Bill Snyder. Note: "Baby Martha" not only survived infancy, she grew up, completed college at Duke University with a degree in computer science, married, had children, and went to work in the computer industry. Today she is a healthy adult; Mildred T. Stahlman, "Assisted Ventilation in Newborn Infants," in *Neonatology on the Web*, 1980. http://www.neonatology.org/classics/mj1980/ch15.html.

11. Mildred Stahlman.

12. As with any "first," there is some controversy about which medical center had the first NICU. Various authorities attribute the first NICU to Stahlman's operation at Vanderbilt. In any case, she is universally considered one of the early pioneers in the field. During the period when she was founding the NICU at Vanderbilt, ground-breaking work in neonatology was also being carried out in Sweden, Canada, and South Africa, where scientists were jerry-rigging their own types of ventilators and methods for monitoring babies.

13. William Altemeier.

14. Robert Merrill.

15. William DeLoache. Note: In 1953, DeLoache formed a pediatric practice group in Greenville, South Carolina, with other pediatricians who had trained at Vanderbilt. In tribute to their mentor, they named it the Christie Group. Christie said he'd grant DeLoache permission to use his name as long as they didn't call it the Christie Memorial Group.

16. Mildred Stahlman, personal interview with David Karzon.

17. Dr. Robert Cotton, professor of neonatology, Vanderbilt University Medical Center, personal interview, June 21, 2005.

18. Ibid.

19. Stuart Finder.

Chapter 11

1. Julie Hollabaugh, "Junior League to Keep Home on White Ave.: Plans for New Location Abandoned, State's Program for Treatment of Disturbed Children Not Hindered," *Tennessean*, (January 16, 1962). From the scrapbook of Mary Louise Tidwell.

2. "Junior League Home Honored: Wins National Accreditation for 3 Years," *Tennessean*, (May 20, 1962). From the scrapbook of Mary Louise Tidwell.

3. Personal letter to Dr. John Walley, potentate, from Mrs. Cromwell Tidwell, president of the Junior League of Nashville, April 19, 1963. From the scrapbook of Mary Louise Tidwell.

4. Ibid.

5. John Seigenthaler.

6. Ridley Wills.

7. Alexander Heard, "A Placid Time, 1964–65," *Speaking of the University: Two Decades at Vanderbilt* (Nashville, Tenn., and London:Vanderbilt University Press, 1995), 37–41.

8. Doyle, *Nashville Since the 1920s*, 195.

9. Ibid., 195.

10. Ridley Wills.

11. Bennie Batson.

12. Amos Christie, personal memo to Dr. John Shapiro, chairman of the Department of Pathology, October 22, 1964.

13. Ibid.

14. "Reader's Companion to American History—Medicaid," Houghton Mifflin, http://college.hmco.com/history/readerscomp/rcah/html/ah_058500.

15. George Holcomb.

16. George Holcomb, personal letter to Dr. Randy Batson, dean of Vanderbilt University Medical Center, December 12, 1966.

17. Conkin, *Gone with the Ivy*, 674–676.

18. "Changing Academic Lifestyles," paper by Amos Christie, found in the Vanderbilt University Medical Center Archives.

19. Interoffice correspondence between Randy Batson and members of the executive faculty, November 29, 1966. Found in the Vanderbilt University Medical Center Archives.

20. George Holcomb, personal correspondence to Randy Batson, dean of Vanderbilt University School of Medicine, December 12, 1966. From the personal files of George Holcomb.

21. Joanne Bailey.

22. Bill Carey, "Money from Medicine," *Fortunes, Fiddles & Fried Chicken* (Nashville, Tenn.: Clearbrook Press Publishing, 2004), 351–362.

23. Lisa A. DuBois, "The Thrill of It All," *Vanderbilt Magazine* (Spring 2003), 42.

24. Carey, *Fortunes, Fiddles & Fried Chicken*, 356.

25. Allaire Urban Karzon, wife of David Karzon and professor of law at Vanderbilt University Law School, personal interview, October 17, 2005; Dr. David Karzon, former chairman of pediatrics at Vanderbilt University Medical Center, found in writings in his personal files.

Chapter 12

1. Allaire Urban Karzon, personal interviews, May 24, 2005, and October 17, 2005. In May 2006, the Karzons celebrated their sixtieth wedding anniversary.

2. Diphtheria is an infectious disease that attacks the throat membranes and can lead to damage in the heart and nervous system.

3. Allaire Urban Karzon.

4. Ibid.

5. William Altemeier. Note: Altemeier was sold. He returned to Nashville, where he'd finished his medical school and residency training. He ran the Vanderbilt program in pediatrics at Nashville General Hospital, teaching pediatric house-staff and practicing "wonderful medicine on a shoestring."

6. Bill Carey, "The Colonel & John Jay," *Chancellors, Commodores, & Coeds* (Nashville, Tenn.: Clearbrook Press Publishing, 2003), 247–259.

7. Robert Merrill, *Amos Christie, MD: The Legacy of a Lineman* (Franklin, Tenn.: Hillsboro Press, 2006).

8. Dr. Robert C. Berson, executive director of the American Association of American Medical Colleges in Washington, D.C., personal correspondence to Randy Batson, director of Medical Affairs at Vanderbilt University Medical School, February 22, 1966.

9. James O'Neill.

10. James O'Neill, personal interview with David Karzon, undated.

11. Amos Christie, former chairman of pediatrics at Vanderbilt University Medical Center, personal letter to Dean Randy Batson, January 9, 1968.

Chapter 13

1. Dr. John Chapman, former dean of Vanderbilt University Medical School, personal interview with David Karzon, July 19, 1999.

2. Charles I. Hendler, "Women Scorned, Children's Hospital Born," 2003, http://preserve.bfn.org/hist/essays/child/child.html.

3. Ibid.

4. Ibid.

5. Christie, *As I Remember It*, 17.

6. Carey, *Fortunes, Fiddles & Fried Chicken*, 396; Ridley Wills; Pat Wilson, member of the Board of Trust at Vanderbilt University. Wilson said he and Andrews worked hand-in-hand to get the liquor by the drink legislation passed. "I was praised by some groups and prayed against—by name—in all of the churches!" Wilson recalled.

7. Nelson Andrews.

8. Ibid.

9. David Karzon, personal interview, May 24, 2005.

10. Nelson Andrews.

11. Frances Jackson.

12. Nelson Andrews, personal interview with David Karzon, September 23, 1998. From the personal files of David Karzon.

13. David Karzon, personal interview with Nelson Andrews, September 23, 1998. From the personal files of David Karzon.

14. Ian Burr, former chairman of pediatrics at Vanderbilt University Hospital, personal interview, April 8, 2005.

15. David Thombs, clinical professor of pediatrics at Vanderbilt University Medical Center, phone interview, December 6, 2005.

16. Eric Chazen.

17. Robert Cotton.

18. Ibid.

19. Nelson Andrews, first chairman of the Vanderbilt Children's Hospital, phone interview, November 8, 2005.

20. Dr. John Chapman, formerly the dean of Vanderbilt University Medical School, personal interview with David Karzon, July 29, 1999.

21. F. Tremaine "Josh" Billings, personal interview with David Karzon, October 14, 1998. From the personal files of David Karzon.

22. Allaire Karzon.

Chapter 14

1. David Karzon, early statements in reference to the formation of the Children's Regional Medical Center. From the personal files of David Karzon.

2. Ibid; Interoffice correspondence to Dean Batson from the office of the senior vice chancellor, Vanderbilt University, November 11, 1970.

3. Pat Wilson.

4. Interoffice correspondence to Dean Batson from the office of the senior vice chancellor, Vanderbilt University, November 11, 1970.

5. After the death of *Tennessean* publisher Silliman Evans, his oldest son Silliman Evans Jr. briefly took over the reins of the newspaper until his untimely death a short time later. Whereupon Silliman Sr.'s younger son, Amon Evans, became publisher.

6. Allaire Urban Karzon.

7. Ed Nelson, former board member of the Regional Children's Medical Center at Vanderbilt University Hospital, interview with David Karzon, October 2, 1998. From the personal files of David Karzon.

8. Nelson Andrews, memo to the board members of the Children's Regional Medical Center, November 17, 1970. From the personal files of David Karzon.

9. Libby Werthan, first president of Friends of Vanderbilt Children's Hospital, personal interview, May 4, 2005.

10. David Karzon, excerpted from personal interview with Ed Nelson, October 2, 1998. From the personal files of David Karzon.

11. Stuart Finder.

12. Nelson Andrews.

13. David Karzon, personal interview with Ed Nelson, October 2, 1998. From the personal files of David Karzon.

14. Suzanne Woolwine, chair of the Junior League Home Board, 1970–71, personal interview, April 4, 2005.

15. Liza Lentz.

16. Jeanne Zerfoss, "Children's Care Units to Merge: Junior League Home, VU Medical Facility Eye June 1, 1971," *Nashville Banner*, November 14, 1970.

17. Ibid.

18. Agreement between the Children's Regional Medical Center and the Junior League of Nashville, December 18, 1970. From the personal files of David Karzon.

19. John Seigenthaler.

20. *"Banner to Publish Shrine Tabloid Oct. 2,"* *Nashville Banner*, January 18, 1971.

21. Betty Nelson Burch, personal interview, April 14, 2005.

22. George Watson Jr., "Civitans Volunteer to Aid Tabloid Sale," *Tennessean*, February 2, 1971.

23. "Frontiers Join Tabloid Sale," *Tennessean*, February 10, 1971.

24. David Karzon, interviews with Bernie Sweet, 1972. From the Vanderbilt University Medical Center Archives.

25. Ian Burr.

Chapter 15

1. "The Junior League Home," 15.

2. Suzie Woolwine, former Home Board chair of the Junior League of Nashville, personal interview, April 4, 2005.

3. Irene Wills, former member of the Children's Regional Medical Center Board, personal interview with David Karzon, undated. From the files of David Karzon.

4. Irene Wills, personal interview, April 7, 2005.

5. Minutes of the Executive Meeting of the Children's Regional Medical Center Board, December 8, 1971; minutes of Children's Regional

Medical Center Board, March 1, 1972.

6. Libby Werthan.

7. Linda Christie Moynihan.

8. Joan Bahner, first parliamentarian of the Friends of Children's Hospital, personal interview, November 11, 2005.

9. Libby Werthan.

10. Carole Nelson, first treasurer of the Friends of Children's Hospital, personal interview, June 1, 2005.

11. Linda Christie Moynihan.

12. Alice Ingram Hooker.

13. Membership report, 1972–73 for Friends of the Children's Hospital. From the personal files of David Karzon.

14. Ibid.

15. Minutes of the Children's Regional Medical Center Board Meeting, Wednesday, January 5, 1972. From the personal files of David Karzon.

16. Letter to Pat Wilson and Tom Kennedy from Libby Werthan, president of Friends of the Children's Hospital. From the personal files of David Karzon.

17. Ibid.

18. Peggy Warner, president of the Junior League of Nashville, personal letter to David Karzon, March 12, 1973. From the personal files of David Karzon.

19. Paul Gazzerro Jr., associate vice chancellor for Medical Affairs for Operations and Fiscal Planning, personal letter to Peggy Warner, president of the Junior League of Nashville, April 3, 1973. From the personal files of David Karzon.

20. "Fun and Fund Raising," *Nashville Banner*, December 18, 1970.

21. Susan Brandau, "Eve of Janus Helps Growth of Center," *Tennessean*, December 26, 1971.

22. Jesse Safley, an editor at the *Banner*, was the first chairman of the Friends' Palm Sunday Paper Sale.

23. William Ross, mail clerk in Vanderbilt Mail Services, phone interview, May 12, 2005. "People ask me what was the biggest show I ever did," Ross said. "Well, there was this little boy in bed and he was really paining. But I did my sleight-of-hand show and got him to smile. I always tell people that that's the number one show I ever did in my life!"

24. Joanne Nairon, former director of the Friends of Vanderbilt Children's Hospital, personal interview, April 26, 2005.

Chapter 16

1. Mildred Stahlman, "Dr. Mildred Stahlman, Oral History," VUMC videotapes 1–3, Culver Productions, October 2, 2002.

2. Robert Cotton.

3. Ibid.

4. "Angel History," http://vuneo.org/history.htm.

5. Carole Nelson.

6. Mildred Stahlman, "Dr. Mildred Stahlman, Oral History."

7. Mildred Stahlman, personal interview with David Karzon, undated.

8. "Proposal for Development of a Division of Pediatric Intensive Care," from the Vanderbilt University Medical Center Archives.

9. Jean Cook, mother of Mollie Wilkerson Cook, phone interview, December 12, 2005.

10. In today's terms, that would translate to $1 million plus in donations.

11. Bill Cook, father of Mollie Wilkerson Cook, phone interview, November 28, 2005.

12. Ibid., phone interview, December 19, 2005.

13. Ibid.

14. Sue Segrest, interoffice memo to Dean Batson and Vice Chancellor Elliott. Subject: "Meeting with the Cooks," December 11, 1968.

15. Ian Burr.

16. Thomas Graham.

17. Harris Riley, from manuscript, "The Karzon Era." From the personal files of David Karzon.

18. Ibid.

19. John Lukens.

20. Ibid.

21. Thomas Graham.

22. Allaire Urban Karzon, October 17, 2005.

23. William "Bill" Bell, former academic specialist representing Ross Pharmaceuticals, phone interview, August 18, 2005.

24. David Thombs.

25. William Altemeier.

Chapter 17

1. John Seigenthaler.

2. "Howard H. Baker Jr. Biography," The University of Tennessee, http://bakercenter.utk .edu/bakerbio.html.

3. John Seigenthaler.

4. Alice Ingram Hooker.

5. "Tomorrow's Votes?" staff photo by Jimmy Ellis, *Tennessean*, November 22, 1973; "Health Care Tour," staff photo by Charles Warren, *Banner*, November 22, 1973.

6. Joanne Nairon.

7. Minutes, Development Committee, Children's Hospital Board, May 4, 1977. From the personal files of George Holcomb.

8. Region VI Junior League Regional Conference invitation. From the personal files of Mary Louise Tidwell.

9. Frances Preston, former president of the Nashville-based offices of BMI, phone interview, November 1, 2005.

10. Mary Frank King, "Ticket Buys Evening of Fun," *Tennessean*, February 17, 1974.

11. Carole Nelson.

12. Ibid.

13. "Recliner Chairs Given Hospital," July 6, 1974; "Children's Fund Expenditures, July 1, 1973 through June 30, 1974." From the personal files of George Holcomb.

14. Ed Nelson.

15. Carole Nelson.

16. Minutes, Development Committee, Children's Hospital Board, May 4, 1977. From the personal files of George Holcomb.

17. Frances Preston.

18. Alice Ingram Hooker.

19. Doyle, *Nashville Since the 1920s*, 92.

20. 2005 Iroquois Steeplechase, "About the Races," http://www.iroquoissteeplechase.org/html/ conditions.html.

21. Alice Ingram Hooker.

22. Mary Stahlman Douglas.

Chapter 18

1. Frances Hardcastle, former treasurer of the Junior League of Nashville, personal interview, April 20, 2005.

2. Frances Hardcastle, personal interview with David Karzon, July 21, 1999. From the personal files of David Karzon.

3. Decree M.B. 82 p. 136, Chancery Court of Davidson County, Tennessee, July 6, 1970, in the matter of *Third National Bank in Nashville, Executor of the Estate of Ora M. Foster, deceased v. Mrs. Ruby M. Pinkerton, et al.*, unpublished, in private collection; decree, Chancery Court of Springfield, Tennessee, March 8, 1965, in the matter of *Earl Farmer, Executor of the last will and testament and estate of C. C. Woodson, deceased v. G. H. Brown, et. al.*, unpublished, in private collection.

4. Decree No. 913, Chancery Court of Cannon County, Tennessee, July 10, 1977, in the matter of *J. H. Larimer, Executor and Meddie Cary, Executrix of the estate of Virginia A. Charter, deceased v. The Imperial Council of the Shrine of North America, whose principal offices is in Chicago, Illinois, and the Shriners Hospitals for Crippled Children, a Colorado Corporation; Vanderbilt University; Nashville, Tennessee; and the Junior League of Nashville, Nashville, Tennessee*, unpublished, in private collection.

5. Woody Sims, phone interview, April 6, 2005.

6. Frances Hardcastle.

7. Decree No. 913, Chancery Court of Cannon County, Tennessee, July 10, 1977.

8. Final Decree No. 77-948-P, Chancery Court for Davidson County, Tennessee, March 10, 1978, in the matter of *Third National Bank in Nashville, under the will of Goodloe Cockrill, deceased v. First American National Bank of Nashville, Executor of the Estate of Sterling B. Cockrill, deceased, et. al.*, unpublished, in private collection.

9. Frances Hardcastle.

10. Transcript of the testimony of Mary Stumb, February 14, 1978, in the case of *Third National Bank in Nashville, Trustee under the will of Goodloe Cockrill, deceased v. First American National Bank of Nashville, Executor of the Estate of Sterling B. Cockrill, deceased, et al.*, No. 77-948-P, unpublished, in private collection.

11. Ibid.

12. Ibid.

13. Ibid.

14. Ibid.

15. Opinion, Court of Appeals of Tennessee, Middle Section at Nashville, June 29, 1979, in the matter of *Third National Bank in Nashville, under the will of Goodloe Cockrill, deceased v. First American National Bank of Nashville, Executor of the Estate of Sterling B. Cockrill, deceased, et. al.* appealed from the Seventh Chancery Division, Part Probate, for Davidson County, Tennessee, unpublished, in private collection.

16. Author's italics.

17. *Third National Bank in Nashville v. First American National Bank of Nashville,* 596 S.W. 2d 824 (1980).

18. Mary Stumb.

19. Frances Hardcastle.

Chapter 19

1. "History of Medicine," Finding Aid to the Vernon E. Wilson Papers, 1953–1981, http://www.nlm.nih.gov/hmd/manuscripts/ead/wilson.html.

2. Frances Meeker, "Vanderbilt's Dr. Wilson Is Man of Many Skills," *Banner,* October 4, 1974.

3. RMP Pre-conference interview with Dr. Arthur E. Rikli, National Library of Medicine, Bethesda, Maryland, interviewer, Storm Whaley, July 25, 1991, http://rmp.nlm.nih.gov/RM/G/G/A/C/.

4. Wayne Wood, "Vanderbilt University Hospital Celebrates 25 Years of Service," *VUMC Reporter* (September 9, 2005), http://www.mc.vanderbilt.edu/reporter/?ID=4202. Note: Jane Tugurian has served as the executive assistant for three vice chancellors of the Medical Center—Vernon Wilson, Roscoe "Ike" Robinson, and Harry Jacobson.

5. James O'Neill.

6. Ibid.

7. Lewis Lavine, former assistant to the vice chancellor for medical affairs, phone interview, December 20, 2005.

8. Pat Wilson.

9. Virginia Keathley, "Driving Force for Hospital," *Tennessean,* August 25, 1976.

10. Lewis Lavine.

11. Ibid.

12. Joe White, "Metro May Get Hospital Wing," *Banner,* August 25, 1976.

13. *Vanderbilt Medicine,* Fall 1988, 21.

14. Sarah Sell.

15. Lewis Lavine.

16. William Altemeier.

17. Allaire Urban Karzon; Conkin, *Gone with the Ivy,* 666.

18. Vernon E. Wilson, personal correspondence to James O'Neill. Subject: "Use of Children's Hospital Beds for Other Services During Times of Low Census," July 13, 1977.

19. Robert Cotton. Note: Cotton said that under Ian Burr's influence the administration changed the way it cost-accounted the NICU to not only take into consideration the revenue from the patient care but the revenue from all the ancillaries. "When all that was done suddenly the NICU became a money winner and the whole attitude toward building a larger unit changed drastically."

20. James O'Neill, personal correspondence to Vernon Wilson, July 1, 1977.

21. James O'Neill, phone interview, December 19, 2005.

22. Frances Hardcastle.

23. Carole Nelson.

24. Ibid.

25. Lewis Lavine.

26. Minutes of New Hospital Liaison Committee—November 29, November 29, 1977.

27. Dr. Vernon E. Wilson, personal correspondence to Ed DiThomas, Minutes of New Hospital Liaison Committee—November 29, December 12, 1977.

28. Alice Ingram Hooker, personal correspondence to John Bihldorff, March 1, 1978.

29. Nancy Humphrey, "The CRS—A Historical Perspective," *Vanderbilt Medicine* magazine (Spring 2003).

30. Ed Nelson.

31. Wayne Wood.

32. Kathryn R. Costello, personal correspondence to Darlene Hoffman, September 23, 1980.

Chapter 20

1. Elise David, "Search to Replace Wilson at Vandy Med Center Set," *Banner*, October 23, 1979.

2. James O'Neill.

3. John Seigenthaler.

4. Mary Lee Manier.

5. Carole Nelson.

Epilogue

1. Liza Lentz.

2. Joanne Bailey.

Bibliography

"About Dr. J. William Hillman." From the Vanderbilt Orthopedic Web page: http://www.mc.vanderbilt
.edu/ortho/hillman1.html.

"Angel History." http://vuneo.org/history.htm.

Armour, Joan. "Tank Town: Its inhabitants: Polio Patients at Vanderbilt." *Nashville Tennessean Magazine* (January 23, 1955).

"Al Menah History." http://www.almenahshriners.org/history.htm.

Carey, Bill. *Chancellors, Commodores, & Coeds*. Nashville, Tenn.: Clearbrook Press Publishing, 2003.

—— *Fortunes, Fiddles & Fried Chicken*. Nashville, Tenn.: Clearbrook Press Publishing, 2004.

A Caring Community: The History of the Jews in Nashville, video. Produced by the Jewish Federation of Nashville and Middle Tennessee.

Christie, Amos. *As I Remember It*. Self-published, 1971.

—— "Early History of Medical Education in Nashville." *Journal of the Tennessee Medical Association* 62 (1969): n.p.

Collins, Robert D. "Troubled Times, 1945–50." *Ernest William Goodpasture: Scientist, Scholar, Gentleman*. Franklin, Tenn.: Hillsboro Press, 2002.

Conkin, Paul K. *Gone with the Ivy: A Biography of Vanderbilt University*. Knoxville, Tenn.: University of Tennessee Press, 1985.

Douglas, Mary Stahlman (with additions). "A History of the Junior League of Nashville."

Doyle, Don H. *Nashville Since the 1920s*. Knoxville, Tenn.: University of Tennessee Press, 1985.

DuBois, Lisa A. "Ernest Goodpasture and the Mass Production of Vaccines." *Lens: A New Way of Looking at Science*. Nashville, Tenn.: Vanderbilt University Medical Center, 2004.

—— "Polio: The Fight Continues." *Lens: A New Way of Looking at Science*. Nashville, Tenn.: Vanderbilt University Medical Center, 2004.

—— "The Thrill of It All." *Vanderbilt Magazine* (Spring 2003): 41–43, 86.

Frank, Feodora Small. *Five Families and Eight Young Men: Nashville and Her Jewry, 1850–1861*. Nashville, Tenn.: Tennessee Book Company, 1962.

—— *Beginnings on Market Street: Nashville and Her Jewry, 1861–1901*. Nashville, Tenn.: Jewish Community of Nashville and Middle Tennessee, 1976.

"General Grant's Infamy." Jewish Virtual Library. http://www.jewishvirtuallibrary.org/jsource/anti-semitism/grant.html.

Halberstam, David. *The Children*. New York: Random House, 1998.

Heard, Alexander. "A Placid Time, 1964–65." *Speaking of the University: Two Decades at Vanderbilt*. Nashville, Tenn. and London: Vanderbilt University Press, 1995.

Hendler, Charles I. "Women Scorned, Children's Hospital Born," 2003. http://preserve.bfn.org/hist/essays/child/child.html.

"History of Children's Hospitals." From the National Association of Children's Hospitals and Related Institutions (NACHRI) and National Association of Children's Hospitals (NACH) Web page: http://www.childrenshospitals.net/Template.cfm?Section=Home&CONTENTID=7418&TEMPLATE=/ContentManagement/ContentDisplay.cfm.

"History of Medicine: Finding Aid to the Vernon E. Wilson Papers, 1953–1981." http://www.nlm.nih.gov/hmd/manuscripts/ead/wilson.html.

"Howard H. Baker Jr. Biography." The University of Tennessee. http://bakercenter.utk.edu/bakerbio.html.

Humphrey, Nancy. "The CRS—A Historical Perspective." *Vanderbilt Medicine Magazine* (spring 2003).

Ingram, Martha Rivers. *E. Bronson Ingram: Complete These Unfinished Tasks of Mine*. Franklin, Tenn.: Hillsboro Press, 2001.

"In the Beginning," adapted from "The Junior League Home" and *The Volunteer* (fall 1981).

"Inventory of the Stahlman, Mildred Thornton (1922–) Collection Number 382." http://www.mc.vanderbilt.edu/sc_diglib/archColl/382.html.

Lewis, John. *Walking with the Wind*. New York: Simon & Schuster, 1998.

Merrill, Robert. *Amos Christie, MD: The Legacy of a Lineman*. Nashville, Tenn.: Hillsboro Press, 2006.

Mid-Missouri Civil War Round Table. "Another Order No. 11: A Near-American Holocaust of 1862." http://www.mmcwrt.org/2001/default0104.htm.

"Mission and History." Children's Hospital of Philadelphia Web page: http://www.chop.edu/about_chop/mission_hist.shtml.

"No Child Is Ever Alone," *Nashville Tennessean Magazine* (January 15, 1950).

Obituary in *The Child*. Home Economics Archive: Research, Tradition and History, "Dr. Horton Casparis, Physician to Children," December 1942. http://hearth.library.cornell.edu/cgi/t/test/pageviewer-idx?c91bd2f4217e2ba702b37721521a4e4&idno=4732639_155_009&c=hearth&view=im.

"Patrick Bouvier Kennedy." http://www.patrick-bouvier-kennedy.biography.ms/.

Pride, Dana. "The Great Divide." *Nashville: An American Self-Portrait*. Edited by John Edgerton and E. Thomas Wood. Nashville, Tenn.: Beaten Biscuit Press, 2001.

RMP Pre-conference interview with Arthur E. Rikli, National Library of Medicine, Bethesda, Maryland. Interviewer, Storm Whaley. July 25, 1991. http://rmp.nlm.nih.gov/RM/G/A/C/.

"Shrine History." *Pyramid Shriners*. http://www.pyramidshriners.com/history.htm.

"The Shrine of North America." http://shrineauditorium.com/shriners.html.

"Shriners Hospitals for Children." http://www.shrinershq.org/shc/lexington/index.html.

Silverman, Mark, T. Jock Murray, Charles S. Bryan, eds. *The Quotable Osler*. Philadelphia, Penn.: American College of Physicians, 2003.

Simmons, John. *The Scientific 100: A Ranking of the Most Influential Scientists, Past and Present*. New York: Citadel Press, 1996.

Slate, Billy J. "Nashville on the High Seas." http://pages.prodigy.net/nhn.slate/nh00032.html.

Snyder, Bill. "Intensive Caring: Stahlman Has Always Demanded Excellence from Herself, Others." *Reporter*, Feb. 4, 2005.

Stahlman, Mildred T. "Assisted Ventilation in Newborn Infants." In *Neonatology* on the Web, 1980. http://www.neonatology.org/classics/mj1980/ch15.html.

———— "Dr. Mildred Stahlman, Oral History." VUMC videotapes 1–3, Culver Productions, October 2, 2002.

Stuart, Hattie, ed. "The Junior League Home." Nashville, Tenn.: Junior League of Nashville, 1983.

Summerville, James. *Nashville Medicine: A History*. Birmingham, Ala.: Association Publishing Company, 1999.

"The *Tennessean*," http://www.answers.com/main/ntquery?tname=the%2Dtennessean&print=true.

Tennessee Blue Book, 2001–2004 (online version). http://www.state.tn.us/sos/bluebook/online/bbonline.htm.

2005 Iroquois Steeplechase. "About the Races." http://www.iroquoissteeplechase.org/html/conditions.html.

Waddle, Ray. "Days of Thunder: The Lawson Affair." *Vanderbilt Magazine* (fall 2002).

Wood, Wayne. "Vanderbilt University Hospital Celebrates 25 Years of Service." *The Reporter*, September 9, 2005. http://www.mc.vanderbilt.ed/reporter/?ID=4202.

Index

Bold indicates photos and italics indicate chapter quotes.